Manual for IV Therapy Procedures & Pain Management

Manual for IV Therapy Procedures & Pain Management

Fourth Edition

Shila R. Hayden, RN,BS,MS,PhD

Copyright © 2009 by Shila R. Hayden, RN,BS,MS,PhD.

Library of Congress Control Number:		2009903460
ISBN:	Hardcover	978-1-4415-2709-7
	Softcover	978-1-4415-2708-0

This book was printed in the United States of America.

To order additional copies of this book, contact:
Xlibris Corporation
1-888-795-4274
www.Xlibris.com
Orders@Xlibris.com
47082

CONTENTS

PREFACE

Intravenous therapy continues to evolve into an ever increasing role within the healthcare field. New technology, expanded patient care settings and aggressive therapies have created vast opportunities and increased responsibilities for personnel performing I.V. Therapy procedures. I have attempted to address the major areas relating to I.V. Therapy as well as the additional areas of growth and expansion in new IV access devices, pain management, care of immunosuppressed patients, home care and care for the caregiver in a practical and easy format.

Any invasive procedure breaks down the body's natural defense mechanisms and is a potential cause of infection. It is the responsibility of everyone involved in IV therapy to understand the care of the patient requiring intravenous therapy, the infusion site and equipment. It is equally important to recognize danger signals and take measures to prevent problems that can arise with patients and their infusion systems. Therefore, this manual presents guidelines to the principles as well as the practice of IV therapy and infection control. Patients generally seek medical help because of disease processes or the presence of pain. In addressing the needs of the total patient these entities must be addressed as well as the technical aspects of acquiring and maintaining intravenous access. The care of patients is a physical, emotional and psychological drain on the caregiver and without appropriate recognition and subsequent attention to the stressors perpetuated upon him/her the caregiver can become exhausted and ineffective in their ability to continue providing quality care.

PUBLISHER'S NOTES

Shila R. Hayden RN,BS,MS,PhD brings to this guide a wealth of education and experience in intravenous therapy, infection control, home care, pain management and stress interventions. She is currently President of Life Link Associates, Inc., a nursing education and consulting company and a Clinical Educator for Bayhealth Medical Center in Dover, Delaware. She was formerly the Director of Patient Care Services and Pain Management Specialist at Good Samaritan Hospital in Baltimore, Maryland, Director of Metcare Pharmacy, Director of Infusion Therapy with Technicare Pharmacy, Consultant for Manor Care, Inc., Administrator for the Care Group Home Care agency in MD, Administrator for Apria Home Care in MD, Director of Woodhaven Pharmacy Infusion Services, Director of infusion services at the University of California, Davis Medical Center in Sacramento, California, Vice President of Nursing at River View Hospital in California, and supervisor of the IV Therapy Department at Sinai Hospital, Baltimore, Maryland.

She has also been a faculty member of Howard County Community College, Essex Community College and Baltimore County Community Colleges in Maryland. She was on the staff at the American River College in California and the University of Central California. She has served as instructor in IV Therapy for the Harford County and Cecil County (Maryland) volunteer ambulance corps and the Emergency Medical Technicians program in California, and has taught the principles and practice of IV therapy and pain management to numerous RNs, LPNs, nursing students, paramedics, and technologists.

In addition to her other responsibilities, Dr. Hayden has served as chairman of the Standards Committee of the National Intravenous Therapy Association (1977-1978), president of the association's Chesapeake chapter (1978-1979), vice president of the Northern Maryland Association of Practitioners in Infection Control (1978-1979), and president of the Sacramento Valley Chapter of NITA (1983).

Dr. Hayden was admitted to Sigma Theta Tau (national honor society for nurses) in 1983, and that same year was honored and presented with an award by the University of Central California for her contribution to excellence in medical education for the state of California.

In 1985 Dr. Hayden established the IV program at the Visiting Nurses Association in Baltimore, Maryland and directed its IV Therapy program. Assuming the position of Vice-President with Care Consultants, a Home Care Nursing Company, in 1989, Dr. Hayden provided training and program development for IV and pain management for patients in the home care setting.

ACKNOWLEDGMENTS

My deepest love and appreciation go to my children, Deborah, Donna and Daniel and to my partner Mary McLaughlin for their love, patience and support in making this fourth edition a reality. Gratitude also goes to those listed below for their contributions and assistance in making this a practical and effective manual:

Nabil Musallam, MS RPh, University of California, Davis Medical Center, Sacramento, California, for critiquing of and additions to Chapters 13, and 15.

Cynthia Mather BS, RN, my friend and colleague, at Bayhealth Medical Center, for her excellent work in taking the photographs for this edition. Her support and encouragement will always be remembered.

CHAPTER 1

A. PURPOSES OF IV INFUSION

- ➤ Administer medications, especially those needed to take effect quickly
- ➤ Supply nourishment, fluids, and electrolytes to body tissues
- ➤ Restore blood volume and correct deficiencies in blood components
- ➤ Stimulate the circulation in cases of shock and vascular collapse
- ➤ Maintain a line to the venous circulation of the patient
- ➤ Measure central venous pressure and blood gases if arterial blood is not available
- ➤ Provide a pathway for anesthetics
- ➤ Obtain blood specimens (phlebotomy)
- ➤ Provide venous access for diagnostic exams (IVP, scans, etc.)

B. CHOICE OF METHOD

There are three basic ways to enter a vein. Choice depends on IV devices available, specific indications for use of the IV, the condition of the patient's veins, the length of intended therapy and the training/expertise of the individual initiating the line.

1. Cutdown is surgical exposure of a vein. It is done when no surface veins are available for entry with a needle. The catheter is threaded directly into the exposed vein.

2. Catheter-through-needle (CTN) Central Lines

These devices are used to enter large veins such as the subclavian, jugular, femoral, basilic, median basilic, or cephalic veins (see Figure 1-1). They are generally utilized for:

o   Long term infusion therapy
o   Total Parenteral Nutrition
o   Vesicant drugs
o   Medications with a high osmolarity

3. Catheter-over needle (CON) and winged needle-Peripheral Lines

The catheter-over-needle (CON) and winged needle (Figures 1-2 and 1-3) are used to enter peripheral veins. Peripheral venipuncture is by far the most common technique. It involves less trauma to patients, is less likely to create problems, is more convenient, and takes less time than a CTN or a surgical cutdown. There are two types of CON's:

a. **Short (¾"-2 ½"):** These are used for short term peripheral venous access and are changed every 48-72 hours.

b. ***Long (3"-8"):*** These are used for longer term peripheral venous access and are changed less frequently than the short catheters. The interval of time at which they must be changed is dependent upon the material the catheter is made of (consult the manufacturers recommendations).

c. ***Special advantages of the CON.*** With this device, the needle is entirely removed and disposed of after venipuncture. Because a catheter is flexible, not rigid like a needle, and no sharp needle is left in the vein, the risk of complications is greatly reduced, especially if the patient is active. Another advantage: The puncture in the vein is exactly the same size as the catheter, since the catheter enters the vein over the needle. This reduces the possibility of blood or fluid leakage around the venipuncture site. A CON is generally preferable to a winged needle.

d. **Special advantage of the winged needle.** With improvements in materials and manufacturing methods, this device is being increasingly supplanted by the CON. However, a winged needle is still preferred when it is necessary to use a very short or small vein, or to administer an IV push or subcutaneous drug.

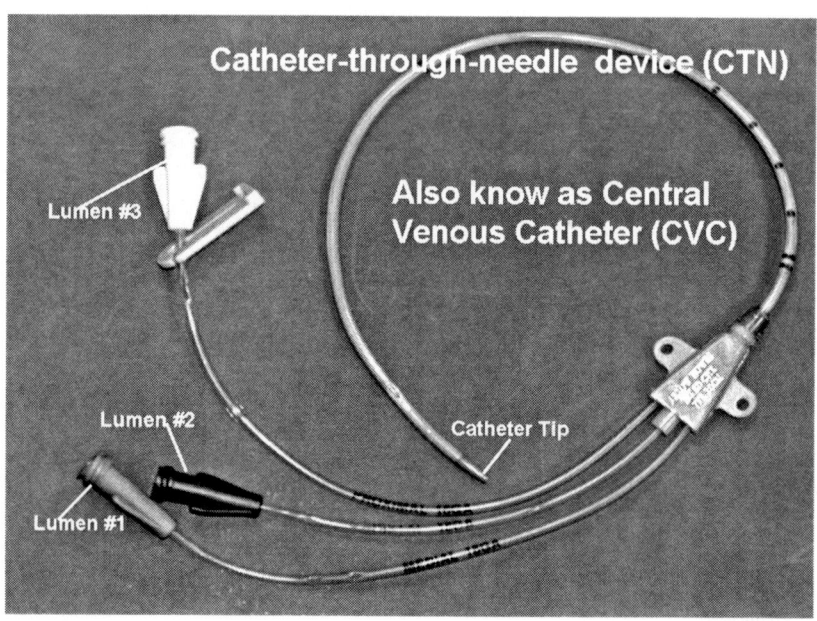

Figure 1-1. Catheter-through-needle (CTN) device

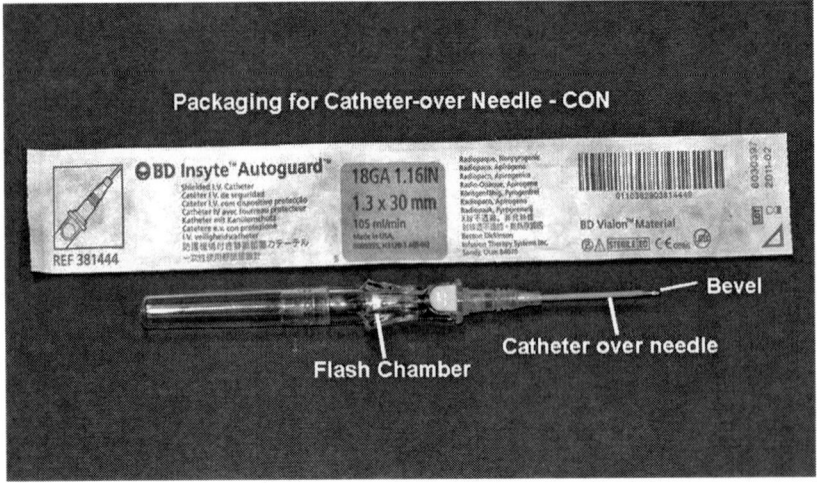

Figure 1-2. Catheter-over-needle (CON) device

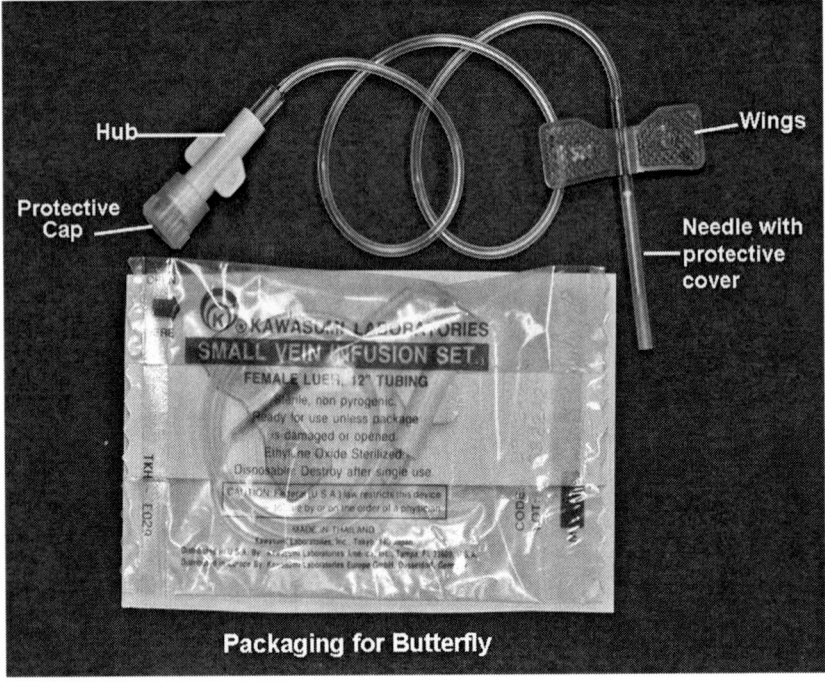

Figure 1-3. Winged infusion set

C. ASEPTIC TECHNIQUE

Whether a vein is entered by cutdown, by CTN, CON or winged needle, except in critical emergencies, aseptic technique must be used in preparing, inserting and maintaining the infusion system.

CHAPTER 2

The Circulation

Veins present the most accessible route for parenteral therapy and nutrition because they are abundant and easy to locate. Knowledge of the anatomy and physiology of veins and arteries will give you a sense of discrimination in choosing veins and help decrease trauma to patients.

A. THE CIRCULATORY SYSTEM

The body's circulatory system has two main subdivisions: cardiopulmonary and systemic.

1. The cardiopulmonary system

This system is not used for intravenous therapy, but it is helpful to review the anatomy since what happens in the systemic circulation may directly affect the cardiopulmonary circulation. Blood enters the heart through the superior and inferior venae cavae and empties into the right atrium. Next it flows through the tricuspid valve into the right ventricle, then through the pulmonary artery to the lungs, where it discards its waste, carbon dioxide (CO_2), and picks up oxygen (O_2). The blood returns through the pulmonary vein to the left atrium of the heart and then flows through the bicuspid valve to the left ventricle. From the left ventricle it enters the aorta, beginning its journey through the systemic circulation.

2. Systemic circulation

This system, especially the peripheral vessels, is used in IV therapy.

a. ***Direction of circulatory flow.*** The aorta—the largest vessel—ascends from the left ventricle of the heart. The aorta branches into arteries, which in turn branch into arterioles, or small arteries. The arterioles branch into capillaries, which are thin walled and permeable for exchange of gases (O_2 for CO^2) and nutrients. Venules—the smallest veins—collect blood from capillaries and deliver it to the veins. Veins bring blood back to the heart's right atrium. To keep blood flowing up toward the heart, veins contain many one-way valves.

b. ***Pressure.*** Pressure in veins is lower than in arteries because veins do not have the benefit of the heart's pumping action—hence the need for valves.

c. ***Elasticity.*** Arteries have more elastic fibers than do veins. These fibers help the arterial walls to withstand the high pressure of the blood that is pumped through them. As there are fewer elastic fibers in the lining of the veins than in the lining of the arteries, veins can constrict or dilate more readily. A distended vein, because it is less elastic, will not resume its shape as quickly as an artery.

B. STRUCTURE OF ARTERIES AND VEINS

The walls of both arteries and veins consist of three main layers (see Figure 2-1).

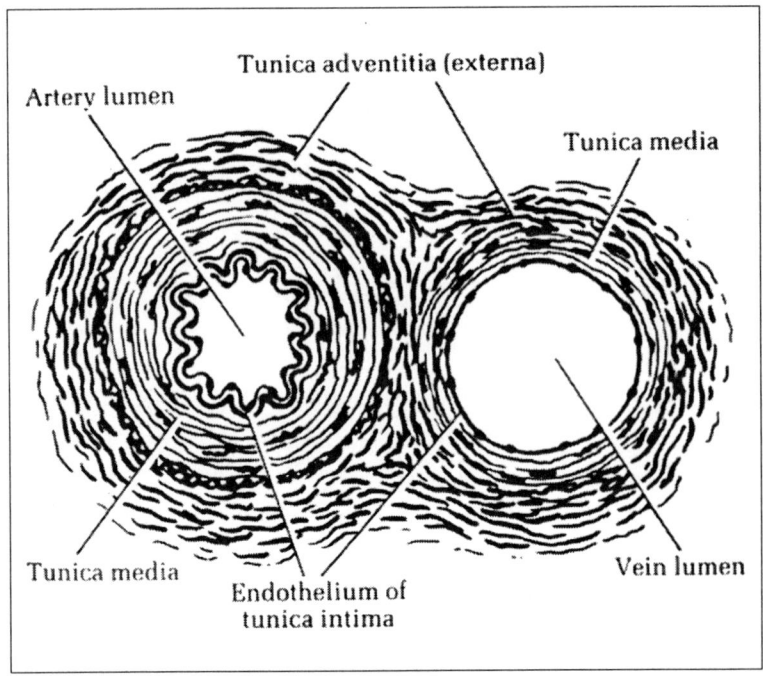

Figure 2-1. Cross sections of medium-sized artery and vein, showing the tunica intima, tunica media, and tunica adventitia (externa) x 250.

1. Tunica intima

   a. Composition. This innermost layer consists of endothelium, which is made up of smooth flat cells. Because it is smooth, blood cells and platelets can flow freely through the Lumen. When inserting and removing needles and catheters, be careful not to scratch or roughen this inner surface by unnecessary movement of the device in the vein. Cells and platelets may accumulate in rough places and form a thrombus. The thrombus may eventually block circulation in the vessel or may break off, creating an embolus.

   b. Valves. Arteries do not have valves; veins do. Valves are semilunar folds in the endothelial lining. They occur most often in the extremities and at points of branching. Sometimes they cause veins to bulge. Avoid venipuncture just below bulges, as you may otherwise hit and damage a valve.

2. Tunica media

  a. ***Composition.*** This middle layer consists of muscle, elastic tissue, and nerve fibers. The vasoconstrictors and vasodilators Located in this lining permit the veins to contract or dilate in response to various stimuli, such as heat, cold, or drugs. As noted before, this layer is thicker in arteries than in veins.

  b. ***Spasms.*** Spasms of veins are due to infusion of cold fluids too quickly, to chemical irritation by a drug, to mechanical irritation, or to strong emotional stimuli, such as fear. They can be relieved by applying heat, which dilates the vein and promotes the flow of blood, by calming the patient, or by removing the source of stimulation causing the irritation. Spasm of a vein is less serious than spasm of an artery. Arterial spasm may block circulation, resulting in necrosis and gangrene, if not relieved promptly.

3. Tunica adventitia (tunica externa)

  a. ***Composition.*** This outer layer consists of areolar connective and elastic tissue. It is thicker in arteries than in veins.

  b. ***Function.*** Its primary function is to hold the vessel together. As people age, the body's connective tissues, including the outer layer of their veins, becomes thin. This thinning process makes their veins extremely fragile, accounting for frequent and easy bruising.

C. SUPERFICIAL VEINS OF THE UPPER EXTREMITIES

Each person has a distinctly individual venous network available for peripheral IV infusion. While many of the major veins may be the same, individual variations are expected in peripheral circulation. Figure 2-2 shows the superficial veins of the dorsal aspect of the hand. Peripheral and central veins of the upper body can be seen in Figure 2-3.

1. Digital veins

The dorsal digital veins run along the sides of the fingers and are joined by connecting branches. They can be used when other veins are not available and will accommodate a small-gauge winged needle or 22- or 24-gauge CON. When utilizing the digital veins for IV infusions, be sure to tape the device securely in place and properly support it to prevent movement of the joint. A tongue blade may be used as a splint for a specific finger, or a hand board may be applied to support the entire hand.

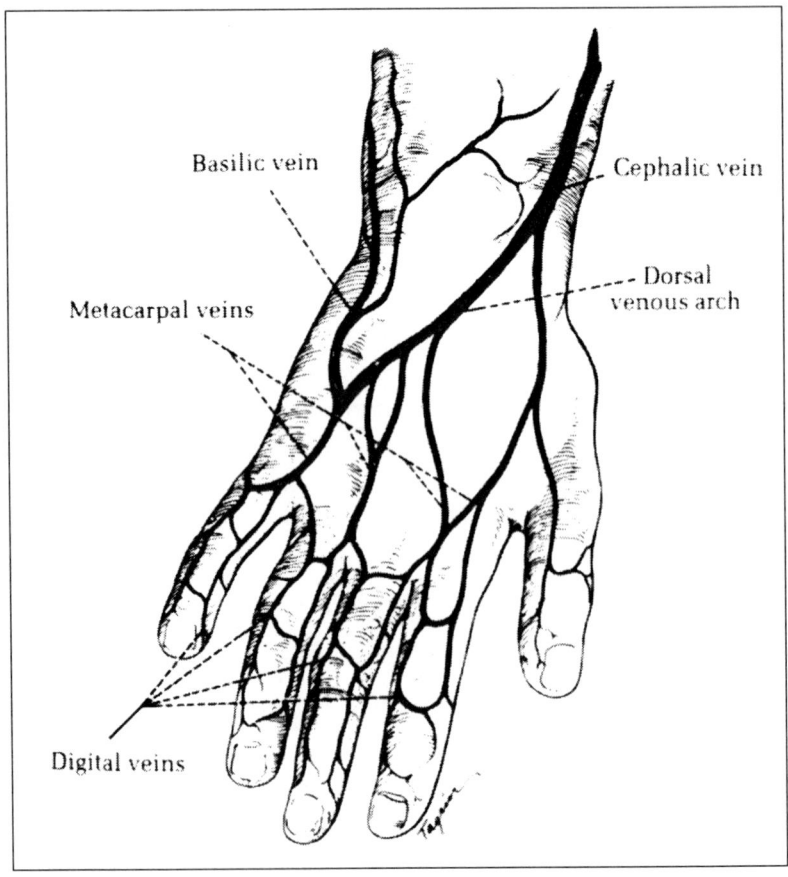

Figure 2-2. Superficial veins of the dorsal aspect of the hand

Reproduced, with permission, from Plumer AL: *Principles and Practice of Intravenous Therapy*, 3rd ed. ©1982, Little, Brown and Company.

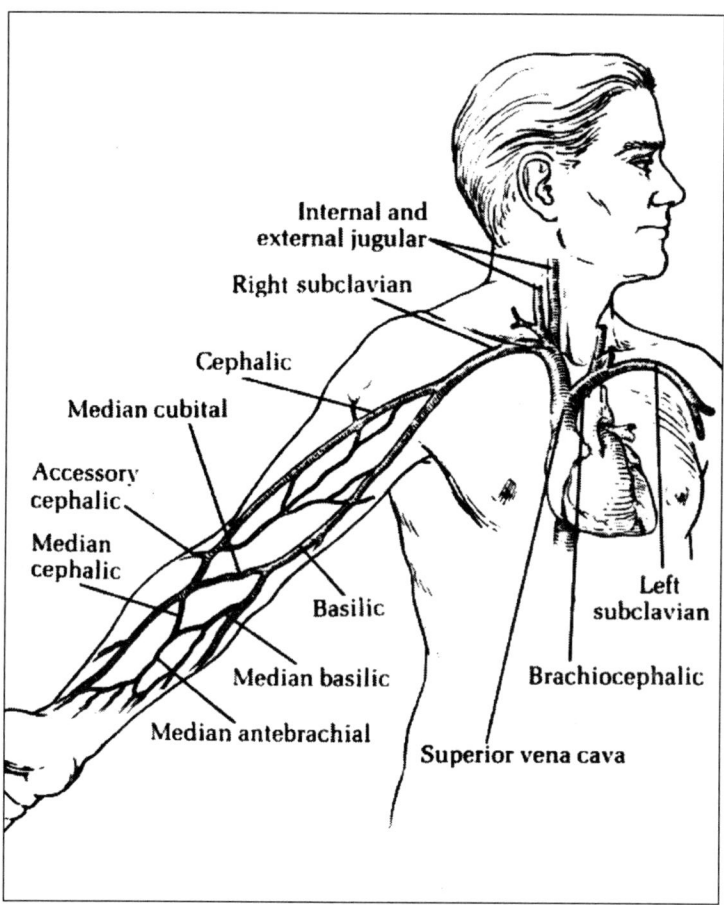

Figure 2-3. Peripheral and central veins of the upper body

2. Metacarpal veins

a. ***Location.*** These veins are formed by union of the digital veins on the back of the hand and include the metacarpal veins, which make up the dorsal venous arch. They are ideal for IV use: They are usually visible, they lie flat on the back of the hand, and the metacarpal bones act as a splint for the IV device.

b. ***Venipuncture.*** In a normal adult, the metacarpal veins are usually the first to be used. Start venipuncture at the most distal point on the extremity. Subsequent venipunctures can then be made above the previous site. This is especially important if the previous site is irritated, phlebitic, or infiltrated.

c. **Elderly patients.** Take extra care with elderly patients. Their skin and vessels are often very thin and the tissue and muscle support is inadequate. This may make them especially susceptible to fast-forming hematomas.

d. **Support.** Firm, secure taping is always necessary. In most cases, use a hand board.

3. Cephalic vein

a. **Location.** The cephalic vein runs upward along the radial border of the forearm, sending branches to both surfaces of the forearm as it goes. It provides an excellent route for IV infusion: It is often visible, it readily accommodates large (low-gauge) catheters or needles, and the radius provides a natural splint.

b. **Venipuncture.** The cephalic vein may be entered from the wrist area to the upper arm—always using the most distal site first. A hand board is necessary when the IV is located in the wrist area.

4. Accessory cephalic vein

a. **Location.** The accessory cephalic vein originates from a plexus on the dorsum of the forearm or from the dorsal venous network. It often branches off from the cephalic vein just above the wrist and rejoins it near the elbow. The accessory cephalic readily accepts large catheters or needles and is an excellent choice for transfusions and IV infusions.

b. **Venipuncture.** The accessory cephalic vein may be entered anywhere along its course, but the most distal site should be used first.

5. Basilic vein

a. **Location.** The basilic vein originates in the ulnar portion of the dorsal venous network and ascends the ulnar surface of the forearm. Just below the elbow it curves toward the inside of the forearm and meets the median cubital vein. The basilic may be entered anywhere along its course, above as well as below the antecubital fossa.

b. ***Venipuncture.*** Because it is inconspicuous, the basilic vein is often overlooked. Always look and feel for it when you are having trouble finding a suitable site. Flex the patient's elbow, so the catheter points in the direction of venous flow, to start the IV infusion.

6. Median antebrachial vein

a. ***Location.*** The median antebrachial vein arises from the dorsal venous plexus, runs along the ulnar side of the forearm, and empties into the basilic or median cubital vein. It is not always easy to find.

b. ***Venipuncture.*** The median veins are not generally desirable for IV infusions because they lie near large numbers of nerves, arteries, and other structures. They should be considered as last resorts for infusions into the upper extremities.

7. Median cephalic and median basilic veins

a. ***Location.*** These veins are found in the antecubital fossa and are generally used for drawing blood or insertion of a midline catheter (4" to 8") or a peripherally inserted central line catheter (PICC).

b. ***Infusion.*** If either of these veins must be used for the insertion of a short CON or winged needle (as a last resort or in an emergency situation), the elbow must be immobilized with a long arm board. This may cause pain and stiffness to the elbow joint. A CON or winged needle started in this area should be changed as soon as possible to a more suitable location. In case a hematoma begins to develop while initiating an infusion in the antecubital area, do not flex the patient's elbow to attempt to stop the bleeding. Apply digital pressure over the site with a sterile gauze pad and raise the patient's arm until the bleeding stops.

D. ARTERIAL PUNCTURE

Inadvertent puncture of an artery may occur if proper insertion technique is not observed or in two anomalous situations: arteriovenous anastomosis and aberrant arteries.

1. Arteriovenous anastomosis

An arteriovenous anastomosis is a direct opening between an artery and a vein. The vein is therefore filled with high pressure arterial blood.

   a. **Causes.** Anastomosis may be congenital, it may be caused by an accidental simultaneous puncture of an adjacent artery and vein, or it may be surgically created (to produce an AV shunt).
   b. **Venipuncture.** The vein will look unusually large, firm, and tortuous, and will appear to be a good vein. It will pulsate due to the presence of arterial blood. This is readily detected when the vessel is palpated. When it is pierced, the blood will come out in spurts. You will have difficulty threading a catheter against the force of the blood. Repeated punctures will prove unsuccessful, painful, and injurious to the lining of the vein. If IV tubing is attached, fluids will not flow freely but blood will back up into the tubing toward the solution because of the high pressure of arterial blood.
   c. **What to do.** Withdraw the catheter/needle, apply pressure over the site with a sterile gauze pad for at least five minutes, or until the bleeding stops, and then try another site.

2. Aberrant arteries

Aberrant arteries are arteries that are located superficially where they are not expected, or where you may expect to find a vein. They are frequently seen in thin or emaciated persons and often occur bilaterally. Their incidence is approximately 1 in 10 persons.

   a. **Cause.** Aberrant arteries are congenital.
   b. **Venipuacture.** The artery will pulsate, which may be felt when the vessel is palpated. When it is punctured, blood will

spurt and will enter a syringe under its own power without aspiration. You will have difficulty threading a catheter. If you do succeed in threading the catheter, the blood will continue to advance up the tubing. The blood will be bright red, not the darker venous hue.

c. ***What to do.*** Withdraw the catheter/needle, apply pressure over the site with a sterile gauze pad for at least five minutes, or until the bleeding stops, and try another site. Do not use the same site on the patient's other side, as you may hit a contralateral aberrant artery.

CHAPTER 3

The Skin

The skin is important in IV therapy because you must pierce it in order to reach any vein. Familiarity with the skin's thickness and consistency at various venipuncture sites will enable you to pierce it correctly and prevent perforation and infiltration. Proper cleansing of the skin at venipuncture sites (see Chapter 7) is also important, as any organisms present there can enter the patient's circulation via the catheter/needle. The skin consists of two main layers—the epidermis and dermis—and overlies the superficial fascia (see Figure 3-1).

A. *EPIDERMIS*

The epidermis, or top layer of skin, is composed of horny (squamous) cells that are relatively insensitive. It is the body's first and main line of defense against invasion by microorganisms.

1. Thickness

The epidermis is thickest on the palms of the hands and soles of the feet and thinnest on the inner surfaces of the extremities. Thickness also varies with age and physical condition.

2. Catheter/needle insertion

The angle of insertion will be more perpendicular to the skin where the epidermis is thicker and closer to the skin where the epidermis is thinner.

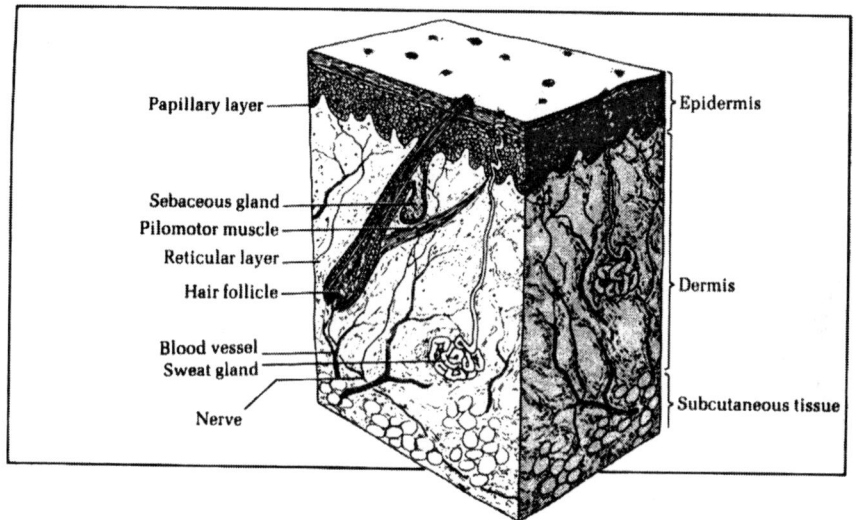

Figure 3-1. Three-dimensional view of the skin

Reproduced, with permission, from Chaffee EE, Greishimer EM: *Basic Physiology and Anatomy*, 3rd ed. Philadelphia: J.B. Lippincott Company, 1974

B. DERMIS

The dermis lies directly under, and is much thicker than, the epidermis. The dermis houses blood vessels, hair follicles, sweat and sebaceous glands, small muscles, and nerves.

1. Thickness

The thickness of the dermis varies on different parts of the body and is also dependent on age and physical condition.

2. Sensitivity

Because the skin is an organ of touch, it contains many small blood vessels and afferent nerves and is highly sensitive. It reacts quickly to temperature, touch, pressure, and painful stimuli. The number of nerve fibers varies in different parts of the body, so that some areas are more sensitive than others.

3. Catheter/needle insertion

Most of the pain associated with starting an IV infusion occurs in the heavily innervated, highly vascular dermis. Therefore, insert your catheter/needle through these two layers as quickly and smoothly as possible.

C. SUPERFICIAL FASCIA

The superficial fascia consists of subcutaneous fibroareolar connective tissue. It lies below the epidermis and dermis, Provides a covering for the blood vessels, and varies in thickness. It is found over almost the entire surface of the body connecting the skin with the deep or aponeurotic fascia. As infection in the tissue of the superficial fascia spreads easily throughout the body, it is very important to use careful aseptic technique for insertion and maintenance of IV devices.

CHAPTER 4

Shock

When starting an IV line in an emergency, remember that most traumatically injured people are in some sort of shock.

A. DEFINITION OF SHOCK

Shock occurs when the pumping action of the heart is insufficient in maintaining the flow of blood through the vessels. As a result, the peripheral vessels constrict and the circulatory pattern shifts in order to sustain the supply of oxygenated blood to vital organs, especially the heart, lungs, kidneys, and brain. The degree of constriction depends on the degree and type of shock

B. TYPES OF SHOCK

The list below contains only some of the many different types of shock.

> ➤ Hypovolemic—due to loss of fluid through hemorrhage (internal or external), burns, vomiting, diarrhea, or severe hyperglycemia in diabetics
> ➤ Neurogenic—due to peripheral vascular dilation as a result of nerve stimulation or nerve block, as in spinal cord injuries
> ➤ Cardiogenic—due to failure of the heart to pump sufficient blood

> Respiratory—due to lack of inspired oxygen, as in narcotic overdoses or drug-alcohol interactions
> Septic (or toxic)—due to widespread infection or poisoning
> Psychogenic—due to overwhelming emotion, such as fright (including fear of injection)
> Anaphylactic—due to allergy to a drug or foreign protein

C. RECOGNITION OF SHOCK

Constriction of the peripheral vessels produces several characteristic signs:

> Pallor of skin, lips, eyelids, gums, tongue
> Cool, moist skin, often beaded with cold sweat
> Rapid breathing
> Hypotension and widening pulse pressure
> Weak, rapid, thready pulse
> Anxiety, clouded senses, disorientation
> Low urinary output and/or thirst

D. TREATMENT

Treatment of shock is based on several principles, but it must be prompt and appropriate to the cause and degree of shock.

1. Open airway

Maintain an open airway and support respiration. Failure to keep the airway open is the most common cause of death in shock patients.

2. Stop hemorrhage

Locate accessible external hemorrhage sites. Apply compression dressings to reduce fluid loss.

3. Cardiopulmonary resuscitation

Preserve normal cardiac and respiratory function by applying CPR as needed.

4. Volume replacement

   a. **IV fluids.** These include lactated Ringer's solution, saline, dextrose, serum albumin, plasma protein fraction, dextran, packed red cells, and fresh frozen red cells; whole blood is now rarely used. Chapter 19 discusses these fluid preparations and their compatibility in more detail.

   b. **Trendelenburg position.** Raising the lower extremities increases the blood supply to the heart, lungs, kidneys, and brain. However, because this position pushes the abdominal viscera up against the diaphragm, reducing the patient's breathing capacity, some now recommend elevating only the patient's feet.

   c. **Inflatable antishock trousers.** These appliances, by constricting the legs and lower abdomen, increase the blood supply to vital organs. They should only be applied, or removed, by personnel specifically trained in their proper use.

E. SEVERITY AND COMPLICATIONS

1. Slight degree of shock

   a. An average deficit of 1 liter of blood or a blood pressure 20% below normal.
   b. It is reversible.

2. Moderate degree of shock

   a. An average deficit of 1.8 liters of blood or a blood pressure 35% below normal.
   b. It is also reversible if treated promptly.

3. Severe degree of shock

   a. An average deficit of 2.5 liters of blood or a blood pressure 50% below normal.
   b. It is an acute condition that may progress rapidly to irreversibility and death.

4. Disseminated intravascular coagulation

    a. ***Definition.*** Disseminated intravascular coagulation (DIC) is a clinical condition manifested by an imbalance in the body's blood coagulation system. It is the result of an underlying disease process. Blood begins to clot within the peripheral circulation, followed by excessive, diffuse fibrinolysis.

    b. ***Cause.*** DIC may be activated by injury to the body's tissues, red blood cells, or endothelial cells. Some common events that may precipitate the DIC process include heat stroke, near drowning, cardiac arrest, septicemia, extensive burns, major chest trauma or surgery, hemorrhage, cancer of the lung or prostate, leukemia, obstetrical accidents, chemotherapy, snake bites, and major organ failure.

    c. ***Recognition and treatment.*** DIC may vary from obscure internal bleeding to mild oozing from the skin, GI tract, GU tract, or wound, to profuse hemorrhaging. It may begin insidiously or suddenly. Blood loss should be carefully measured and blood replacement should be an integral part of the therapy. Treatment should be aimed at alleviating the underlying cause and should be supported by use of appropriate drugs and intravenous fluids. It is vitally important that DIC be recognized rapidly and treatment initiated promptly if serious consequences, including possible death, are to be prevented.

F. THE PATIENT IN SHOCK

Always treat shock seriously. It can progress rapidly from a slight state to one that is irreversible. Remember to treat any life-threatening condition that may be present first, then initiate IV therapy. Intravenous fluids will increase the circulatory Volume and help decrease the effects of shock. Do not say anything in front of an unconscious patient that you would not say if the person were conscious. The patient may only appear to be unresponsive. Remember: The sense of hearing is the last to go.

CHAPTER 5

Selecting And Preparing The Equipment

NOTE: IV infusions started in emergency situations outside a hospital setting are usually initiated under less than aseptic conditions. These IV lines should be changed to a new site once the patient is admitted to the hospital to minimize the possibility of infection.

A. BASIC EQUIPMENT

1. IV solutions (sterile)

A variety of IV solutions are utilized according to the patient's needs. These solutions and their functions can be found in Chapter 19 under the heading "Types of Fluids". IV solutions may come in glass bottles, plastic bags or semi-rigid containers.

2. Administration set (sterile)

The standard/straight administration set includes the following parts:

- Spike
- Drip chamber
- Tubing
- Regulator clamp
- Injection ports (tubing may or not have these ports)
- Adapter/end connector
- Protective cap

3. Catheter/needle devices (sterile)

The type of device you use for venipuncture depends on several considerations:

- Purpose of infusion (medication, anesthesia, hydration, nutrition, etc.)
- Size of peripheral vein selected
- Patient's age and condition of their veins
- Nature of infusion (continuous, intermittent, one-time bolus)
- Length of anticipated therapy

> NOTE: For therapies that will last for several weeks it may be more advantageous to select a long peripheral catheter (Midline) rather than a short peripheral catheter that needs to be changed more frequently. The patient's peripheral venous access, the length of therapy and the specific infusate need to be considered when choosing this method. TPN, Chemotherapy, Vesicant and irritating medications should be administered through a central line and not a peripheral or Midline catheter.

- Number of simultaneous infusions anticipated.

> NOTE: For infusions of more than one IV fluid/medication at the same time, a double lumen peripheral (Twin Cath manufactured by Arrow, Int.) or multi-lumen central line catheter should be selected. This will help to decrease the number of punctures and trauma to the patient's veins or possible interaction of incompatible fluids/medications.

a. CON Choices:

> ➢ 12,14, or 16 gauge X 1 ½ or 2 inches (or longer)for multiple major trauma, infusing large amounts of blood or fluid quickly under pressure, and for extensive surgical procedures, transplants, cardiac surgery, etc.
> ➢ 18 gauge—x 1 ¼ TO 2 inches—for major trauma, major surgery, cardiac arrest, or blood transfusions.

➢ 20 gauge—X 1 ¼ to 1 ½ inches—for minor trauma, minor surgery, blood transfusions, and cardiac arrest when unable to insert an 18 gauge catheter.

➢ 22-gauge x 1 inch—for routine Keep-vein-open (KVO) infusions, pediatric patients (with medical problems), and for most medical needs.

➢ 24-gauge x ½ or ¾ inch—for infants or when necessary to start an infusion in a digital or scalp vein or a small, spidery vein; never to be used when any type of surgery is indicated.

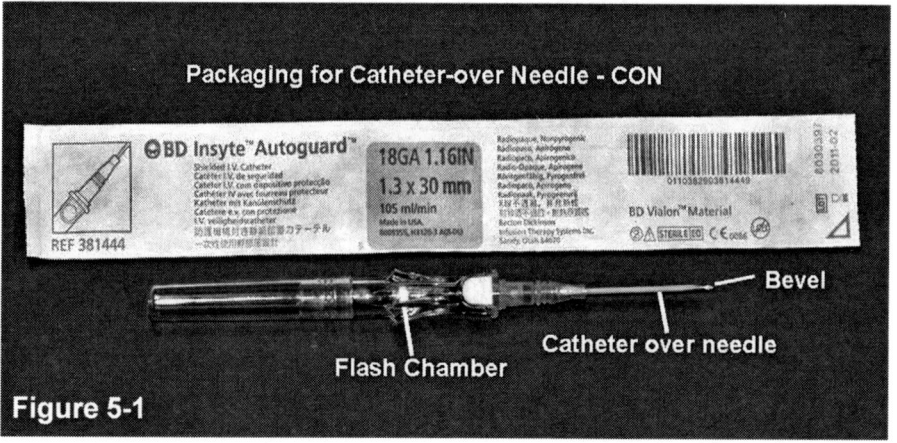

Figure 5-1

b. *Parts of a CON:*

➢ Bevel tip
➢ Needle/stylet
➢ Catheter
➢ Flash chamber
➢ Syringe or vented plug
➢ Hub
➢ Protective cap

c. *Winged needles.* Use these sizes for entry into veins for infusions of short duration or when the patient is allergic to the materials used in the CON device:

➢ 19-gauge—comparable to a 18-gauge CON

- ➢ 21-gauge—comparable to a 20-gauge CON
- ➢ 23-gauge—comparable to a 22-gauge CON
- ➢ 25-gauge—comparable to a 24-gauge CON—used for small, spidery veins or for neonates, if you cannot insert a CON
- ➢ 27-gauge—smaller than CON's—used for extremely small veins

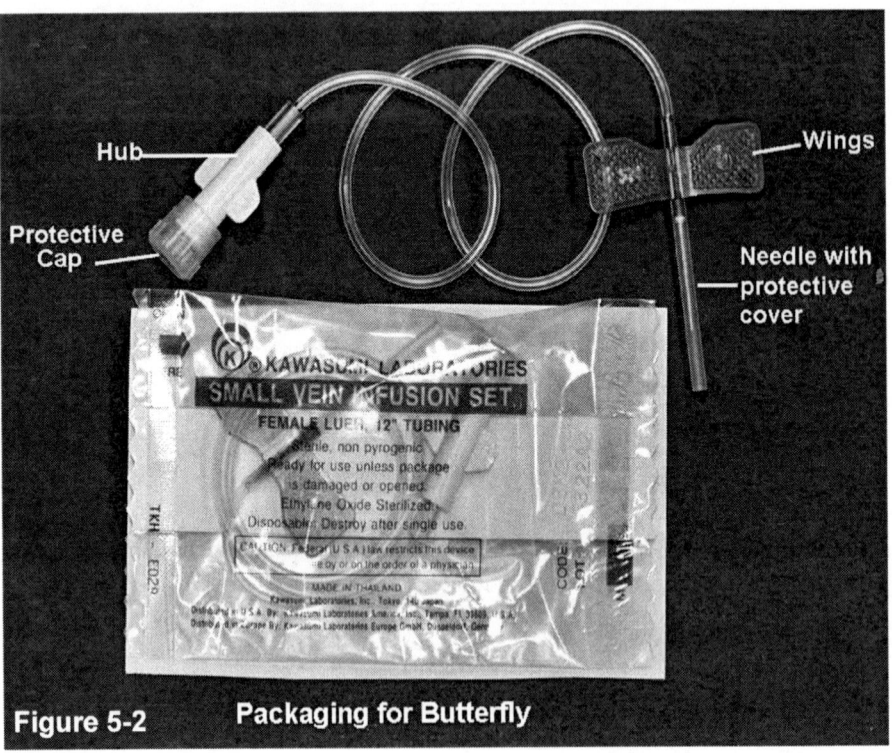

Figure 5-2   **Packaging for Butterfly**

4. Tourniquet

5. Paper, Dermicel, or Transpore tape

NOTE: Do not use adhesive tape. It is extremely hard on a patient's skin.

6. Arm board

- ➢ Short—for the hand or wrist area

> Long—for IVs located in the antecubital fossa (unless a midline or peripherally inserted central catheter (PICC) is utilized that will not kink)

7. Dressing:

> Dry gauze sponge (2 x 2)
> Band-aid
> Transparent dressing

8. Alcohol wipes and a povidone-iodine wipe or a Chlorhexidine (Chloraprep®) for cleansing the anticipated puncture site.

NOTE: Because it is often impossible to obtain an allergy history in an emergency situation, povidone-iodine wipes should not be used on patient's when their allergy status is unknown.

9. IV pole or hooks

B. ADDITIONAL EQUIPMENT

1. CTN device (Central Lines)

The catheter-through-needle devices are generally inserted in the subclavian, jugular or femoral by a physician or the the basilic, median cubital or cephalic veins by a physician or specially trained Registered Nurse. These catheters may remain in place for longer periods of time resulting in fewer venipunctures for the patient. They are primarily used for total parenteral nutrition, vesicant medications and solutions or medications with a high osmolarity.

2. Midline catheter

This is a long line catheter (approx. 3-8" in length) that is generally inserted in the basilic, median cubital or cephalic vein just above or below the antecubital fossa. The entire catheter remains in the peripheral vasculature. This catheter may remain in place for longer periods of time than the traditional short (1-2") catheter resulting in fewer venipunctures for the patient. The amount of time a

Midline may remain in place is determined by the manufacturers recommendations and facility policy and procedures.

3. Twin-Cath*

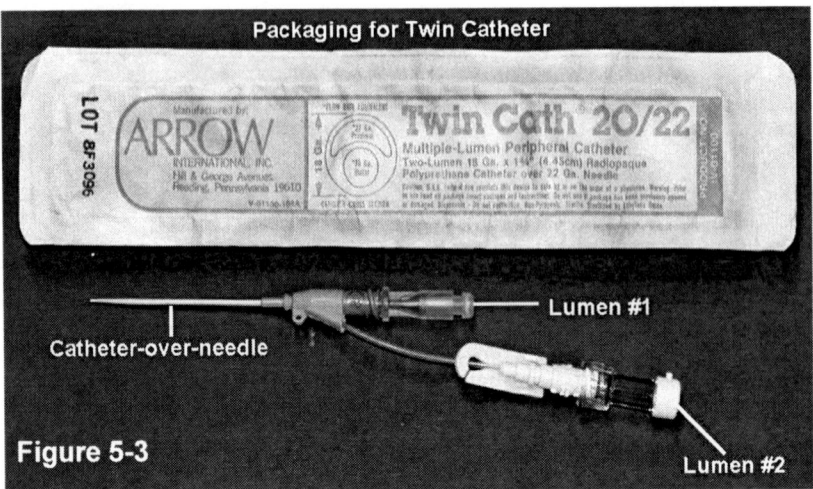

Figure 5-3

This is a double lumen peripheral catheter. The double lumen feature of this catheter allows incompatible fluids to be infused simultaneously through the same peripheral line.

4. Vented tubings

Vented tubings should only be used with unvented glass bottles. Plastic bags automatically contract as they empty, so the flow is unimpeded without the need for venting.

5. IV tubing with macrodrip chamber

Macrodrip IV tubings are available in three sizes:

- 10 drops/ml (see figure 5-4)
- 15 drops/ml (see figure 5-4)
- 20 drops/ml (see figure 5-4)

☐   Twin-Cath: Manufactured by: ARROW International, Inc. Reading, PA

6. IV tubing with microdrip chamber

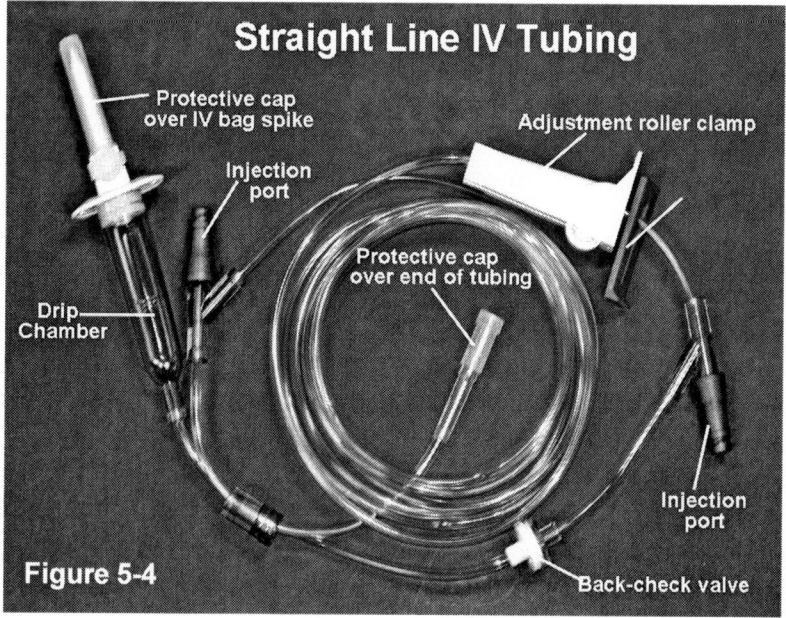

Straight Line IV Tubing

Protective cap over IV bag spike

Adjustment roller clamp

Injection port

Protective cap over end of tubing

Drip Chamber

Injection port

Figure 5-4

Back-check valve

Microdrip chambers deliver 60 drops/ml and are used for various purposes:

> ➤ To deliver small amounts of medication over long periods of time
> ➤ To regulate the flow of medication very precisely
> ➤ To keep a vein open

7. Filter

Filters come in various pore sizes:

> ➤ 1 to 5 microns—removes only large particulate matter and no bacteria
> ➤ 0.45 micron—removes all particulate matter and some bacteria
> ➤ 0.22 micron—removes all particulate matter and all bacteria, fungi, and yeasts

8. Gravity-feed piggyback set

A piggyback is a secondary set used for intermittent drug administration. It runs into the upper Y port of the primary IV line. Because the piggyback container must hang higher than the primary container, in order for the infusion to run by gravity, an extension hook is provided for the primary bottle/bag.

9. Simultaneous infusion

A second IV tubing may be attached to the lower Y port of the primary line for simultaneous infusion of a second fluid. Both containers of fluid may hang at the same height.

10. Volume-control chamber

A volume-control set, or fluid chamber, is used to deliver small amounts of medication diluted in precise quantities of fluid. It may be used as the primary set for an infant or small child, or for an adult requiring precise measurements of fluids and/or medications. Because a volume-control chamber is easily contaminated (by frequent injections into the system), a piggyback setup is generally preferred whenever possible.

11. Stopcock

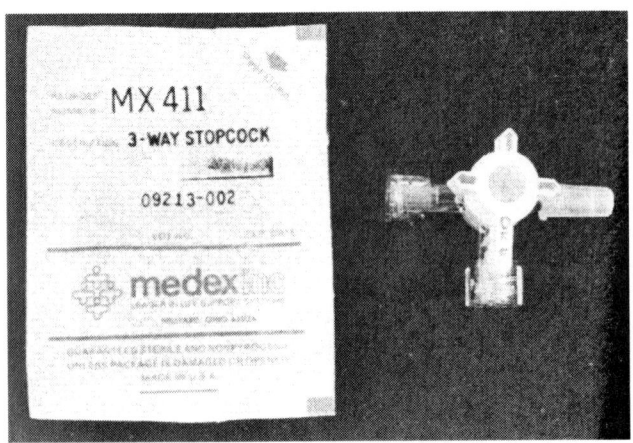

Figure 5-5. Stopcock

A stopcock (see Figure 5-5) may be added to an IV line to provide for direct injection of a medication.

NOTE: Whenever a stopcock is added to an IV line, extra care must be taken to ensure that the ports remain covered and that the entire infusion system does not become contaminated.

12. Dressings

The following types of dressings may be used:

> ➢ Sterile gauze pad (2 x 2)
> ➢ Band-Aid (sterile)
> ➢ Transparent film (sterile)

13. Blood transfusions sets

There are several types of transfusions sets:

> ➢ Straight-line set with built-in blood filter—for whole blood, packed red cells, frozen cells, or washed cells
> ➢ Y set—when saline is needed, as with packed red cells or whole blood through a secondary line
> ➢ Microaggregate filter set—for large amounts (more than three units) of packed red cells, frozen cells, or washed cells; also for immunosuppressed patients or those with potential febrile leukocyte reactions
> ➢ Component syringe set—for platelets or cryoprecipitates when infusing by IV push
> ➢ Component drip set—for platelets or cryoprecipitates when infusing by IV drip

When large quantities of blood must be administered quickly, extra equipment is needed:

> ➢ Transfusion pump—either built-in or slip-on
> ➢ Blood warming device—immersible coil or electric warmer

14. Intermittent-infusion reservoir (PRN adapter)

There are several types of adapters that are used to create an intermittent line which allows the patient to maintain mobility:

- ➢ Standard heparin lock (winged infusion device)
- ➢ Adapter plug used with standard needle
- ➢ Adapter plug with flexible CON (see Figure 5-6)
- ➢ Latex seal attached to CON device
- ➢ No-needle reservoir systems (see Figure 5-6)

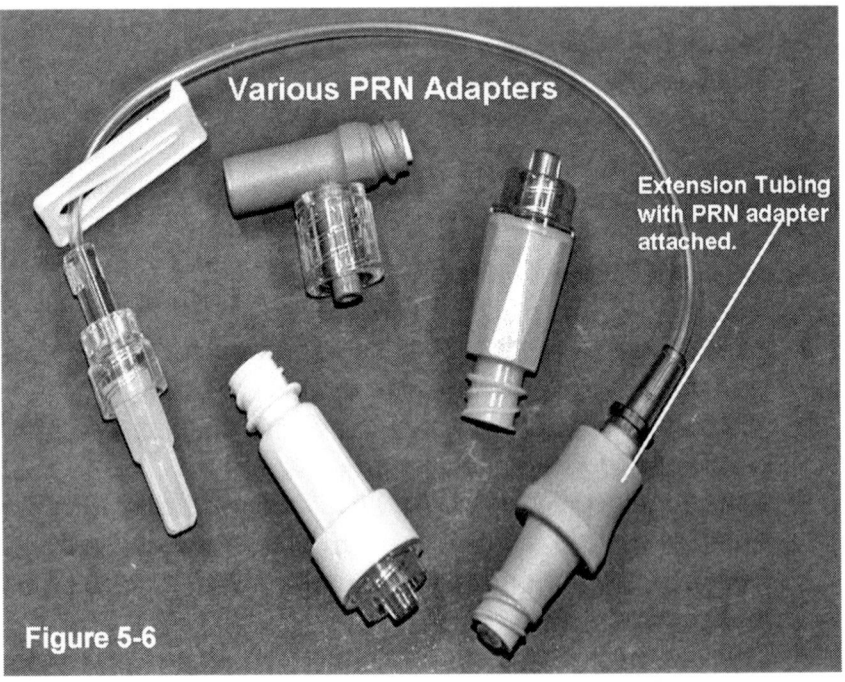

Figure 5-6

PRN adapters may be used on any peripheral or central line for intermittent infusions. Positive pressure prn adapters are beneficial since only saline needs to be used to flush and maintain patency of the catheter.

Note: All adapters may be used with a saline and/or heparin flush.

15. Infusion pumps and controllers

Various types of pumps and controllers are available and serve a variety of needs:

> Syringe pumps—used for very slow and precise infusions and KVO rates (0.01 ml/hour)
> Peristaltic pumps—move fluid through the tubing with a peristaltic, wavelike motion (most peristaltic pumps will deliver 1 to 300 ml/hour)
> Piston-action (volumetric) pumps—the most versatile deliver 1 to 999 ml/hour)
> Controllers—work by gravity flow. Controllers vary in their delivery ranges (most deliver 1 to 300 ml/hour)
> Elastomeric Infusion Devices—work by constriction of the inner elastomeric portion of the device when the clamp is opened to release the pressure. The flow rate is pre-determined by the size of the device and the amount of fluid put into the device. Elastomeric Infusion Devices do not require height to facilitate infusion (no IV pole is needed). Patient mobility is easily maintained with this device and flow rates are consistent and reliable.

16. Swabs or wipes

- Alcohol
- Povidone-iodine
- Chlorhexidine Gluconate (Chloraprep®)
- Skin protector (eg. skin guard)

17. IV pole (prn)

18. Extension tubing or IV loop

An extension tubing or IV loop may be attached to the end of the catheter/needle device. This helps prevent kinking of the tubing and facilitates tubing changes.

CHAPTER 6

Preparing IV Equipment

Whether you are starting an infusion in the hospital, the patient's home, long-term care facility, or in an emergency situation in the field, always assemble and inspect all your equipment before you touch the patient. Maintain sterile technique.

A. HAND WASHING

Wash your hands vigorously with antimicrobial soap or bactericidal solution before beginning the procedure and before going on to each subsequent patient, whether you are starting an IV line or merely changing bottles, bags, tubing, or dressings, injecting medications into a line, or disconnecting a line.

B. INSPECTING YOUR EQUIPMENT

1. IV solution

Check the bottle or bag carefully for:

> ➢ Cracks, leaks, tightness of seals
> ➢ Cloudiness, discoloration, precipitation
> ➢ Correctness of solution
> ➢ Expiration date

If a solution has turned cloudy, consider it contaminated and do not use it.

2. Catheter/needle

    a. **Catheter.** Discard the device if the catheter is bumpy or torn at the ends.

    b. **Needle.** Does the bevel look perfectly sharp and the shaft perfectly smooth?

    c. **Hub.** Does it lock tightly?

    d. **Size.** Is the size appropriate for the purpose of the infusion?

3. Tubing

    a. **Size and type.** Make sure the tubing is the right length and has the necessary ports, clamps, filters, and other devices.

    b. **Leaks.** As you prime the tubing by running fluid through it to remove air (see section C-5 below), check for leaks, especially around ports and connections.

4. Other devices

Carry out a thorough inspection of each extra device you will be adding to the line.

C. SPIKING AND PRIMING

1. Flow clamp

Slide the clamp up the tubing until it is just below the drip chamber. Close the clamp.

    a. **Roller clamp.** To adjust the rate of flow to the desired flow rate, the roller is rolled up to open the line and down to close the line.

    b. ***Screw clamp.*** To adjust the rate of flow to the desired flow rate, the screw is turned clockwise to close the line and counterclockwise to open the line.

    c. ***Slide clamp.*** When using a slide clamp, the rate of flow cannot be adjusted, only turned on or off. To close the line, the tubing is slid into the narrow end of the clamp; to open the line, the tubing is slid to the wide end of the clamp.

2. Spiking

    a. ***Nonvented bottle.*** Remove the cap and wipe the rubber stopper with alcohol. Remove the cover from a vented spike and push the spike firmly into the stopper.

    b. ***Vented bottle.*** Remove the cap and latex cover. If you do not hear a hiss, the bottle's vacuum has been breached and the solution is contaminated. Discard it. If you hear a hiss, remove the cover from a nonvented spike and insert the spike into the larger of the two holes after wiping the stopper with alcohol.

    c. ***Plastic bags.*** If the bag is the kind with a large port and broad lip, it need not be hung before spiking. The other kind must be hung first. Remove the protective caps from the bag and the tubing spike, and insert the spike into the bag with a twisting motion.

3. Hanging

Hang all solutions a distance of at least 36 to 45 inches higher than the venipuncture site if the IV is to run via gravity.

4. Drip chamber

Gently squeeze the drip chamber until it is about half full of solution This will help prevent air bubbles from forming in the tubing.

5. Priming the tubing

The purpose of priming, or flushing, the tubing is to remove air and any particulate matter from the line. The average tubing contains between 5 and 10 ml of air.

a. ***Vented cap.*** If the tubing has a vented protective **end cap**, prime the tubing by opening the clamp and filling the tubing with solution. Gently tap at any air bubbles. Invert any secondary ports or valves and tap at them to release air bubbles. When the tubing is full and no air bubbles remain, close the clamp.

b. ***Nonvented cap.*** If the **protective end** cap isn't vented, you must remove it to flush the air out. Protect the end of the tubing and the cap from contamination. Hold the end of tubing over a sink or wastebasket, open the clamp, and let the solution run through. Tap away all air bubbles as described above. When no bubbles remain, close the clamp. Replace the cap or cover the end with a sterile cap.

6. Hanging the tubing

Loop the primed tubing over the top of the IV pole to keep it safe while you prep the patient and perform the venipuncture. Be careful to maintain the sterility of the connector (end of the tubing) by keeping it capped until you are ready to connect it to the patient's infusion system.

CHAPTER 7

Preparing The Patient For IV Therapy

A. APPROACHING THE PATIENT

1. Identification

Identify the patient by two identifying descriptors (i.e. name, birth date, S.S.#, etc.). If the patient has an armband check the information on the armband as well.

2. Reassurance

Introduce yourself politely and tell the patient what you are going to do. Ask the patient's cooperation in holding still while you perform venipuncture. As you work, continue to give the patient overt and covert reassurance. Emotional tension may cause venous spasms and make venipuncture more difficult. If the patient is an infant or is combative, it may be necessary to restrain the limb, for stability, prior to performing the venipuncture.

3. Allergies

Unless you are working under emergency conditions, you should check the patient's record for a history of allergies. Find out whether the patient is allergic to:

> ➤ Medications, or items in the solutions you are about to infuse

> Iodine
> Tape

4. Clotting disorders and other conditions

Find out whether the patient has a clotting problem, has been taking anticoagulants or any medications that might be incompatible with the one you're about to give. If the patient is about to have a mastectomy or nephrectomy, or surgery on an arm or hip, make sure you know which side so you can start the IV on the opposite side.

B. SELECTING A VEIN

In selecting a vein for venipuncture, consider the size, condition, and location of veins, the patient's age, medical and clinical status, special tests or procedures the patient is undergoing, and the purpose and type of IV procedure.

1. Size of the vein

Larger peripheral veins are easier to find and enter than smaller veins, and they pose less risk of perforation and infiltration or extravasation.

> *a.* **Shock.** A patient in severe shock may have collapsed veins, making it all the more difficult to find a vein for venipuncture.
> *b.* **Drugs.** Veins may be widened or narrowed by drugs with vasodilating or vasoconstricting properties, respectively.

2. Condition of the vein

> *a.* **Palpation.** Always palpate the extremity before you choose a vein. Often the more visible veins are not as suitable for IV infusion as veins that cannot be seen, but only palpated. Palpate for condition of the vein and also to make sure that you do indeed have a vein and not an artery, aberrant artery, or arteriovenous anastomosis (see Chapter 2).

b. ***Phlebitic or infiltrated area.*** If a vein is phlebitic or the area infiltrated due to a previous IV, restart the IV in the opposite limb if at all possible. If the same limb needs to be used, you must restart the infusion above the phlebitic or infiltrated area to avoid any further trauma or irritation to the veins and/or tissues at the affected site.

c. ***Veins to avoid.*** Avoid veins that are:

> ➢ Tortuous
> ➢ Hardened or scarred from age or previous IV use
> ➢ Sore or inflamed from recent use
> ➢ Filled with bifurcations or large, prominent valves

3. Location of the vein

Chapter 2 outlines the anatomy of the peripheral venous circulation in detail, but locations for venipuncture are listed here for quick review.

a. ***Upper extremities.*** In starting and IV in the upper extremities it is important to understand the purpose of the IV and the anticipated level of patient function. You should always start the venipuncture at the most distal site possible that will be suited for the specific needs of the patient. Therefore, the best veins, in the upper extremities, may be in the hands or in the forearms. Use your critical assessment skills in choosing an appropriate site (eg. if a patient is ambulating with a walker or crutches, stay away from the hands and wrist). Working from possible lower to higher sites:

> ➢ Back of the hand
> ➢ Wrist (outer aspect only)—do not start an IV on the inner aspect of the wrist. If fluids infiltrate into this area the pressure can cause nerve damage to the nerves in that area
> ➢ Outer aspect of the forearm
> ➢ Inner aspect of the forearm
> ➢ Upper arm
> ➢ Antecubital fossa

Use the antecubital fossa for an IV infusion only when no other peripheral veins are available in the upper extremities. The antecubital fossa, however, may be an ideal location for giving injections and drawing blood samples. For IV infusions started in the antecubital fossa with a winged needle device it will be necessary to immobilize the elbow joint with a long arm board to prevent an infiltration of the fluids/medications and prevent damage to underlying arteries and nerves. Prolonged immobilization may cause painful stiffness at the elbow. An IV infusion started in the antecubital fossa should be moved at the earliest opportunity.

b. ***Other parts of the body.*** The jugular, subclavian, and other deep veins are ordinarily reserved for patients with limited peripheral venous access and those requiring a central line for special fluids or medications such as total parenteral nutrition. Tunneled catheters (i.e. Hickman's, Groshong, PORT's, etc.) are general utilized for patients requiring IV therapy for extended periods of time. In infants, the scalp vein is usually preferable. If upper extremity veins are not available the following locations may be considered as a means of last resort:

➢ Feet, ankles, and legs
➢ Scalp

Depending on institutional policy, a physician's order may be necessary to start an infusion in a lower extremity. IV's are generally discouraged from being started in the lower extremities because the peripheral veins in the lower extremities unite directly with the deep veins. This may be a source of potential problem (i.e. thrombophlebitis or embolus) for the patient. Also, many adults have varicose veins and fluid or medication may become "pooled" in these varicosities. Lower extremity veins are also contraindicated in patients with diabetes or peripheral vascular disease. If an IV is started in the lower extremities, it should be watched carefully and removed immediately if any signs or symptoms of swelling, redness or tenderness occur.

   c. ***Side of the body.*** Certain surgical procedures may necessitate that the IV be placed on a specific side:

> ➤ Patients having surgery on an arm or a breast will generally have the IV started on the opposite limb
> ➤ Patients having surgery on a hip, kidney, or lung may generally have the IV started on the surgical side
> ➤ For further clarification or specific instructions concerning which side may be best for starting the IV, you may want to check with the patient's physician or anesthesiologist
> ➤ For medical patients, use the non-dominate arm or hand, if possible

4. Age of the patient

   a. ***Infants.*** To simplify problems of restraint, a scalp vein is usually preferred. When using a scalp vein, point the bevel of the needle down, or towards the infant's face, in the direction of blood flow.

   b. ***Geriatric patients.*** Veins in elderly patients may be hardened, or fragile and easily torn. They're also likely to be more tortuous, a result of sluggish circulation. To prevent unnecessary bruising on these patients be sure to use the direct approach when entering the vein (see Chapter 8) and be careful not to puncture the back or side wall of the vein by using a low angle of entry into the vein.

5. Size of the patient

   a. ***Obese patients.*** The veins of the hand, wrist, or inner forearm may be seen faintly, but they may be difficult to palpate. You may have to increase the angle of insertion of the catheter/needle in order to penetrate the extra adipose tissue.

   b. ***Thin or emaciated patients.*** In especially thin patients, you are likely to see fragile, "rolling" veins under thin, papery skin. You will need to anchor the vein very firmly, lower the angle of insertion of the catheter/needle, and use the direct approach for venipuncture (see Chapter 8).

6. Clinical status of the patient

a. **Injured extremity.** Never start an IV on an injured, sore, bruised or diseased extremity, on the stump of an amputated limb, or on an extremity where the pulse is weak or absent.

b. **Position of patient.** If the patient must lie prone or on one side, your choice of vein is limited to the exposed aspect of his/her body.

c. **Mastectomy.** Start an IV on the side opposite the mastectomy. If the patient has had bilateral mastectomies, check the arms for signs of edema and the presence of pulses. Check with the patient's physician to verify where the IV may be placed safely.

d. **Arteriovenous Anastamosis or shunt.** Start IV's on the arm opposite the one with the shunt. If you must use the same arm as the one with the shunt, go well above the shunt area such as the upper arm. Do not leave the tourniquet on the shunt arm for more than one minute; if possible, perform the venipuncture without using a tourniquet. If you do inadvertently puncture an AV fistula, remove the catheter/needle, elevate the patient's arm, and apply pressure to the site for 10 minutes. Notify the physician. If you need to start an IV in a scalp vein of an infant with an AV shunt, perform venipuncture on the side of the head opposite the shunt. If you use a rubber band, as a tourniquet on the infants head, don't leave the rubber band on the infant's head any longer than necessary, and don't place it directly over the shunt.

e. **Mental state.** Even if a patient is unconscious when you start an IV, you must consider the possibility that he/she may wake up confused and agitated. If this seems likely, restraints should probably be used according to your institution's policy. It may also be necessary to restrain a child who is too young to cooperate.

7. Special tests and procedures

  a. **_Angiograms, arteriograms, and aortograms._** Check
  the patient's chart to see which side is being prepped, and
  start the IV on the opposite side. Since most such patients
  have cardiac and/or circulatory problems, fluid overload is
  especially dangerous. Make sure the patient's nurse knows
  an IV has been started so that he/she can watch the patient
  closely for signs of circulatory overload.
  b. **_Pacemaker insertion (transvenous)._** Always start the IV
  in the arm opposite the pacemaker site. If the IV is in the
  same arm as the pacemaker catheter, it is difficult to watch for
  infiltration, as the arm is completely wrapped during catheter
  insertion. You may consult the physician or radiologist as to
  his/her preference for the left or right side.
  c. **_Pancreatic duct cannulation._** Always start the infusion
  according to the physician's or radiologist's specifications.

8. Purpose and type of IV procedure

  a. **_Irritating substances._** If the patient is to receive fluids
  or drugs that may be irritating to the vein, the size of the
  vein selected and the size of the catheter used is extremely
  important. In general, the larger the vein in relation to the
  catheter/needle, the greater the hemodilution of the fluid
  or medication being administered and the less irritating the
  infusion will be to the intima of the vein. Also, there's less
  chance that a small-caliber catheter/needle will come in
  continuous contact with the opposite wall of the vein, which
  will help to minimize irritation. When choosing the size
  catheter/needle to use always use the smallest size that will fit
  the patient's needs. This will help decrease possible irritation
  and trauma to the patient's veins. When it is necessary to
  infuse high osmolarity or highly irritating solutions, a central
  line should be utilized for even greater hemodilution.
  b. **_Prolonged administration._** If you know that the IV will be
  in place for several days, it is especially important to choose
  a site that affords the patient as much comfort and mobility
  as possible. If you still must place the IV in a movable area

such as the hand or wrist, use a short hand board or long arm board. This will help keep irritation to a minimum, decrease the possibility of infiltration, and prevent damage to underlying arteries or nerves. If an IV is going to be required for several weeks you may want to consider either a midline catheter or a PICC line.

c. ***Intermittent-infusion reservoirs, transfusions, and total parenteral nutrition (TPN).*** These special IV procedures are covered in Chapters 14, 18, and 20, respectively.

C. PREPARING THE SITE

1. Filling the vein

It is not always necessary to use a tourniquet, if the patient has a high blood pressure or if the veins are large and/or tortuous, you may not need to apply a tourniquet.

2. Distending the vein

a. ***Gravity.*** Have the patient hold the extremity lower than the heart. This will slow venous return and fill the distal portion of the vein with blood.

b. ***Milking.*** Rub the patient's arm from the proximal to the distal end prior to applying the tourniquet. This will help move blood down toward the lower portion of the arm and the hand.

c. ***Tourniquet.*** Apply the tourniquet 3 to 4 inches above the anticipated puncture site, without pinching the skin or pulling hair. You can improvise a tourniquet from such items as these:

> ➢ Soft rubber tubing tied with a slipknot
> ➢ A blood-pressure cuff inflated to slightly above diastolic pressure
> ➢ A Velcro strap
> ➢ A Penrose drain

In field emergencies, it is possible to use a rope, necktie, belt, or scarf. Do not make the tourniquet so tight that it restricts arterial flow. You can check this by feeling for the presence of a radial pulse after applying the tourniquet.

d. *Tapping.* Lightly tapping the puncture area after applying the tourniquet will help distend the vein.

e. *Fist clenching.* Alternate clenching and relaxation of the patient's fist will help distend the veins. However, if the IV is to be started in the hand, it is best that the hand be relaxed during insertion of the device.

f. *Releasing the tourniquet.* If venous fill seems insufficient, you may briefly release the tourniquet and then refasten it to trap additional venous blood in the extremity.

g. *Compresses.* If the patient is cold, the veins will be constricted. To help dilate the veins, wrap the entire limb in a warm moist towel heated to a maximum temperature of 105° F. Cover it with a water-repellent wrapping and leave it in place for 15 to 20 minutes.

h. *Sclerosed veins.* Sclerosed veins require very little pressure from a tourniquet. In fact, venipuncture may be easier without a tourniquet if the veins are engorged with high-pressure blood.

NOTE: Sclerosed veins may feel hard when palpated. They are not a good choice for venipuncture because the lumen of the vein has been narrowed and it may be difficult to enter the vein successfully.

i. *Relaxation.* A very tense patient may develop spasms or constriction of the veins. Reassurance is very important.

3. Cleansing the site

If the area around the venipuncture site is exceptionally dirty, cleanse it with soap and water before proceeding.

a. *Chlorhexidine Gluconate.* Apply to the skin in a back and forth scrubbing motion for 30 seconds. Allow to air dry. The antibacterial effect will continue functioning under the IV dressing for up to 48 hours.

b. ***Povidone-iodine***. Apply to the anticipated puncture site, using a firm, circular motion from the center to the periphery of an area about 2 inches in diameter, and allow the solution to remain on the skin **until it is dry**. Do not wipe it off. If the povidone-iodine solution is allowed to remain on the skin, its bactericidal effect will continue functioning under the IV dressing.

c. ***70% Isopropyl Alcohol.*** If the patient is allergic to iodine, and Chlorhexidine Gluconate, you may cleanse the area with 70% isopropyl alcohol for a minimum of one full minute **(60 seconds),** use at least two alcohol wipes. Use a firm, circular, center-to-periphery motion. Allow the alcohol to air dry on the skin before proceeding.

d. Once the site has been prepped, it should not be touched again. If the site is touched again, it needs to be prepped again!

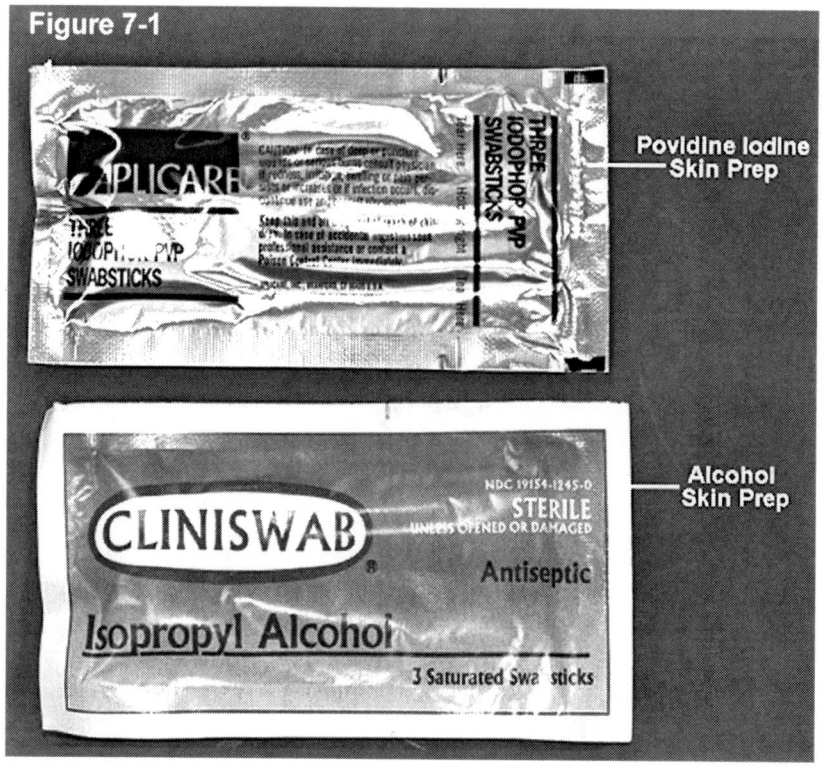

Figure 7-1

Povidine Iodine Skin Prep

Alcohol Skin Prep

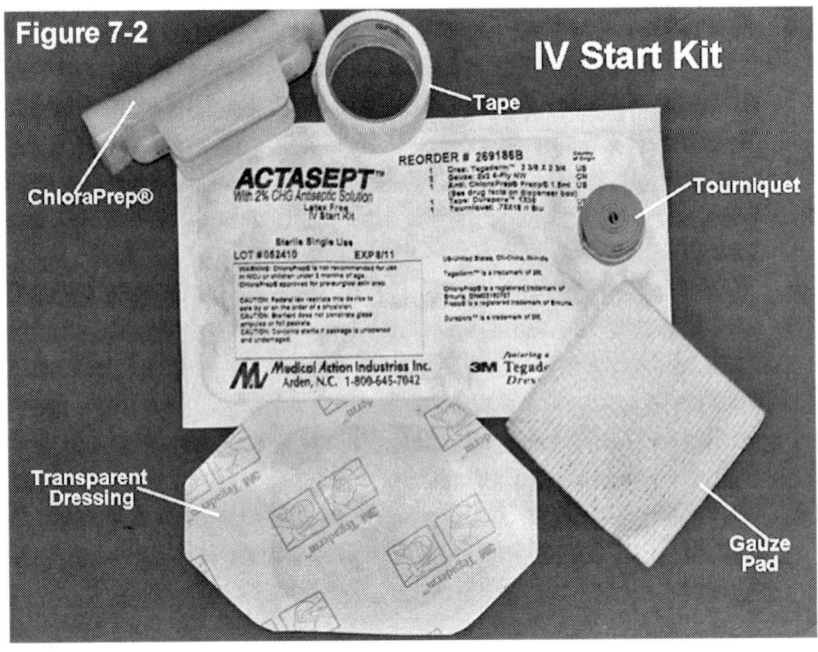

Figure 7-2

IV Start Kit

ChloraPrep®

Tape

Tourniquet

Transparent Dressing

Gauze Pad

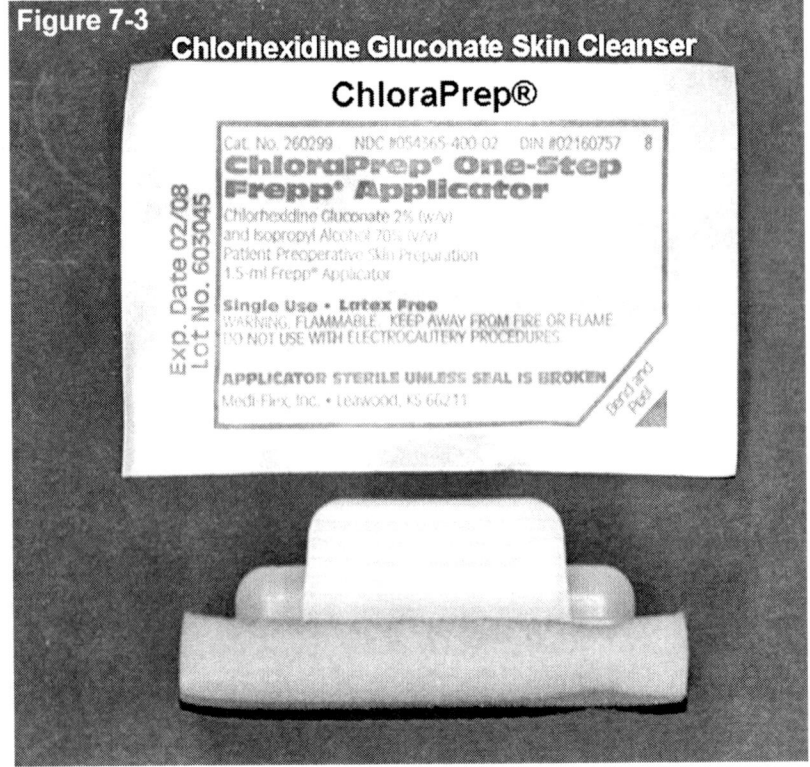

Figure 7-3

Chlorhexidine Gluconate Skin Cleanser

ChloraPrep®

4. Shaving

There is no good evidence for shaving. On the contrary, shaving may be harmful because it produces micro-abrasions that can harbor bacteria. The antiseptic used to cleanse skin is equally effective on hair. However, if the hair around the site is excessively thick, you may:

➢ Clip it with scissors
➢ Back the tape, or place a gauze pad under the tape when securing the catheter in place (see Chapter 9)

CHAPTER 8

Venipuncture technique

A. INSERTION

Maintain sterile technique at all times. Never use a catheter/needle for more than one venipuncture; use a new set up and complete prep for each new puncture. Apply gloves (clean) prior to sticking the patient.

1. Anchoring the vein

With your left hand (if right-handed), hold the patient's arm and stretch the skin in a downward (longitudinal) direction with your left thumb. This stretching tension is important to anchor the vein and keep it from rolling while you insert the catheter/needle. If the vein does start to roll, use firmer tension. Pulling the skin taut will enable the needle to pierce the skin more easily, allowing a non-traumatic entrance into the vein and less pain for the patient. Make sure your left thumb is out of the way of the catheter/needle; if you touch the catheter/needle, it is contaminated and must be discarded.

2. Holding the catheter/needle

    a. **CON.** Grasp the catheter by the clear plastic flash chamber, or syringe, behind the hub. Do not grasp the hub itself; if you do, the catheter may slide down over the bevel of the stylet, damaging the catheter, the patient's skin, and the vein.

  b. **Winged needles.** Grasp the wings. Do not touch the needle itself; if you do, it is contaminated and must be discarded. You may wish to **flush** the winged-needle device with **normal saline** solution prior to sticking the patient.

  c. **CTN.** Check the manufacturer's instructions.

3. Placing the catheter/needle

  a. **Indirect method.** Place the bevel about ¼ inch below, and to the side of, the point where you plan to enter the vein. This method is useful for patients with tough skin.

  b. **Direct method.** Place the bevel directly over skin and vein at the point of venipuncture. This is a useful method for patients with fragile or rolling veins.

4. Piercing the skin

Hold the catheter/needle at a 15 to 45 angle, depending on the texture of the patient's skin (use a sharper angle for tough skin and a lower angle for patients with thin skin). A good general rule is: the thinner the skin, the lower your angle of entry; the thicker the skin, the steeper the angle of entry. Always be sure to warn the patient that you are about to insert the needle, to prevent jumping or flinching due to the element of surprise. Insert the catheter/needle through the skin quickly with a firm, steady motion.

5. Entering the vein

After piercing the skin, lower the catheter/needle slightly and aim directly for the vein. You may sometimes feel a pop when you enter the vein. When blood appears in the flash chamber of the catheter, or the tubing of the winged-needle device, lower the needle even more, until it's almost parallel to the skin. Slowly advance the catheter/needle another 1/4 to 1/2 inch into the vein. If a syringe is attached to the catheter, aspirate to verify good blood return. If there is no syringe attached, slowly advance the catheter according to the manufacturer's instructions. If you are using a winged needle, finish threading the needle up the vein. Release the tourniquet and skin tension and connect the tubing or PRN adapter. Start the infusion according to the ordered rate or flush the line with saline or heparin solution to maintain patency.

6. Threading the catheter

   a. CON. Either of the following techniques may be used:

> **One-hand technique:** While maintaining tension on the skin with one hand, grasp the hub of the catheter and disengage the catheter from the needle or stylet 1/4 to 1/2 inch, with the same hand used to perform the venipuncture. Disengaging the catheter will prevent accidental piercing of the vein with the needle while threading the catheter. Holding the hub of the catheter, advance the catheter up the vein and into position. **You may place a sterile gauze pad under the hub of the catheter to capture any blood that may be leaking out of the hub.** Aspirate once again if the device has a syringe attached. Once you are assured that you have good blood return, verifying that you are still within the vein, release the tourniquet and tension on the patient's skin.

> **Two-hand technique:** Once you have entered the vein verified by a flashback of blood, advance the catheter an additional ¼ to ½ inch. Release the skin tension and use that hand to grasp the hub of the catheter and disengage the catheter from the stylet/needle. Holding the stylet/needle securely with one hand, thread the catheter up the vein and into position with the other hand. Aspirate once again if the device has a syringe attached. Once you are assured that you have good blood return, verifying that you are still within the vein, release the tourniquet.

Note: Both techniques are acceptable. However, the one-hand technique generally realizes a greater percentage of success, especially for the inexperienced. Retraction of the patient's skin when released may be great enough for the vein to draw back off the catheter/needle, causing it to come out of the vein and resulting in an unsuccessful venipuncture. **Additional techniques may be warranted with the introduction of safety catheters/needles. Always refer to the manufacturers directions for safe advancement of the device into the patient's vein.**

b. ***CTN.*** As various types of CTN devices are now available, the manufacturer's instructions should be followed to ensure the proper insertion technique for the specific device. While threading a CTN device, it is very important that you NEVER pull the catheter back through the needle. This could result in a sheering off of the catheter, resulting in a catheter embolus.

c. ***Resistance.*** If you encounter resistance when threading a catheter (either a CON or a CTN), **do *NOT* force the catheter up the vein. You may try loosening the tourniquet to see if that will help with the threading of the catheter.** If that doesn't help, try this procedure:

- Release the tourniquet
- Disengage and remove the stylet
- If there is good blood return, **attach a syringe with normal saline solution or** the primed IV tubing to the catheter
- **Gently flush the vein with the saline solution or** open the clamp and allow the IV solution to flow into the vein
- If no swelling appears and the vein flushes easily or the fluid seems to be flowing, gently try to float the catheter up the vein and into position

Under no circumstances should you reinsert the needle or stylet into the catheter once it has been removed.

7. Removing the stylet

a. ***CON.*** Pull back on the needle and/or activate the safety mechanism—you may press lightly above the catheter tip with a finger. You must see some evidence of blood return. If no blood appears do not connect the IV tubing. The catheter may have become dislodged or perforated the vein. Aspirate again. If you cannot aspirate any blood, withdraw the catheter, discard it, and start over at a new site. If you do see evidence of blood return, you are ready to connect the IV tubing.

b. ***CTN.*** Gently withdraw the needle/stylet and remove it from the catheter per the manufacturers instructions. Continue to thread the catheter to the desired position and tape it securely in place. Place a sterile gauze over the puncture site and cover the site with a sterile dressing **(the gauze dressing should be changed within 24-48 hours to a transparent dressing, without a gauze pad underneath the dressing)**. Connect the catheter to the IV tubing and start the IV infusion, or connect a PRN adapter and flush with the appropriate solution to maintain the patency of the line.

NOTE: The technique may vary according to the CTN device being used. Follow the manufacturer's instructions for each device.

B. COMMON DIFFICULTIES WITH VENIPUNCTURE

Repeated unsuccessful attempts to start an infusion may mean that you need to sharpen you venipuncture skills. **Every time you miss an attempt you need to critique your technique. To improve your technique, become your own worst critic. What didn't you know that you should have known to make the stick successful or what did you do that you shouldn't have done?**

1. Not going far enough into the vein

You may not be inserting the needle far enough into the vein. Remember to advance it ¼ to ½ inch after you have entered the vein. If you are using a CON, the catheter must be well within the lumen of the vein before you can disengage the stylet and thread the catheter.

2. Tension

You may not be maintaining enough tension on the patient's skin, or maintaining tension long enough. Remember to keep the skin taut during the entire procedure.

3. Angle of entry

You may be inserting the catheter/needle at too steep an angle. You may **be going too deep** and perforating the opposite wall of the vein. A good general policy is the thinner the skin the lower your angle of entry into the vein. The tougher, or thicker, the skin the steeper the angle of entry into the vein.

4. Haste

In your desire to spare the patient pain, or to "get it over with" if you're nervous, you may be rushing things. **Remember that it takes a few seconds for the blood to travel from the bevel of the needle/catheter to the flash chamber or tubing. If you are moving too fast you may actually go through the back of the vein before you are even aware that you have entered the vein.** Take your time; it's better for the patient to be stuck only once, the correct way, than to be stuck two or three times **in haste**.

5. Jabbing

You may be jabbing at the vein instead of smoothly sliding the catheter/needle into it.

6. Approach

You may be using an indirect approach when a direct approach is called for (see section A-3 above).

7. When to give up

A common rule of thumb is "Two strikes and you're out" **(although some places may permit three attempts).** Do not make more than three attempts on the same patient, unless it is a life/death situation and you are the only available person. Get someone else—preferably a person with considerable IV experience—to try.

C. USE OF LOCAL ANESTHESIA

1. Personnel

Personnel may be permitted to use 1% plain lidocaine (Xylocaine) intradermally as determined by your institution's policies.

They may include:

- Registered Nurses who have been trained in IV Therapy Procedures
- Physicians

2. *The use of Xylocaine on a routine basis is not recommended as a routine practice.*

This should be reserved for:

A. People who are very frightened and request that it be used
B. Young children who are very frightened
C. Starting a large bore needle (12, 14, 16 gauge)in a conscious patient
D. Starting a Midline or PICC line

NOTE: Never use lidocaine for patients who are allergic to lidocaine or related local anesthetics (e.g., Bupivacaine, Marcaine; Etidocaine, Duranest, Mepivacaine, and Carbocaine).

3. Procedure

- ➢ Wipe the stopper of the vial with alcohol
- ➢ Attach a 25-gauge, five-eighth inch needle to a sterile syringe, or use a tuberculin syringe
- ➢ Draw up 0.5-1ml of 1% plain lidocaine using aseptic technique, and expel all air
- ➢ Apply a tourniquet, select the site for venipuncture, and remove the tourniquet
- ➢ Thoroughly cleanse the area around the site with 70% isopropyl alcohol
- ➢ Insert the tip of the needle into the subcutaneous tissue at a 15 to 30 angle
- ➢ Aspirate; if no blood appears, inject a small amount off lidocaine to produce a small wheal
- ➢ Advance the needle and aspirate again; if no blood appears, inject some more lidocaine to produce a small wheal
- ➢ After injecting the lidocaine, withdraw the needle and gently rub the injection site with a sterile gauze pad. Perform the venipuncture.

If you aspirate blood prior to injecting the lidocaine, stop. Don't inject any lidocaine. Instead, withdraw the needle, gently apply pressure to the site with a sterile gauze pad, and start over at a new site. Don't inject more than 1ml of lidocaine at any time, and always use plain lidocaine **(without epinephrine).**

4. Emla Cream

Emla cream may be applied to the skin to anesthetize the anticipated venipuncture site. It should be applied 30-45 minutes prior to the venipuncture. Once the Emla cream is applied, cover the site with a transparent dressing. When you are ready to perform the venipuncture, remove the transparent dressing and wipe the Emla cream off. Continue with the routine prep and venipuncture.

5. Other products may be used as available and appropriate to numb the anticipated venipuncture site.

Follow the manufacturer's directions for safe usage.

CHAPTER 9

Starting An IV Infusion

A. CONNECTING THE TUBING

1. Adapter

Remove the protective cap from the end of the tubing and connect the tubing to the hub of the catheter or to the prn adapter. Remember to wipe the prn adapter off for 10-15 seconds prior to connecting the IV tubing.

2. Checking the flow

Open the clamp to make sure the IV solution will flow freely.

3. Checking for infiltration

If the area around the venipuncture site becomes swollen or painful after the solution has begun to enter the vein, the solution may be infiltrating the surrounding tissue. If so:

> ➢ Close the clamp
> ➢ Withdraw the catheter/needle
> ➢ Apply pressure to the site with a sterile gauze pad until the bleeding stops. Cover the site with a sterile bandage. Pick a new site and begin the procedure again.

> ➤ Apply warm, moist compresses to the infiltrated area to speed up absorption of the IV solution in the surrounding tissue.

NOTE: If medications or additives to the IV solution would be irritating or damaging to the tissues, you would apply cold compresses to the infiltrated area to slow down the absorption process and decrease the irritation to the tissues.

4. Clamping the tubing

Set the regulator clamp at a slow (KVO) rate while you do the next two steps: cleansing and taping.

B. CLEANSING THE VENIPUNCTURE SITE

1. Blood

With a sterile gauze pad, or alcohol swab, cleanse the area of any blood. Blood is an excellent medium for bacterial growth and must not be left around the puncture site.

2. Antimicrobial ointment

Antimicrobial ointments are not recommended for use on IV sites. If the site has been prepped with the Chlorhexidine, 70% Isopropyl alcohol or povidone-iodine solution and allowed to remain on the skin to dry, no additional applications are necessary.

C. TAPING THE IV DEVICE

All IV devices must be securely taped to the patient's skin. This helps prevent catheter or needle embolism, perforation, dislodgement, and trauma to the inside of the vein. Movement of the catheter/needle inside the vein is not only irritating but also enlarges the percutaneous opening so that bacteria can enter **and greatly increases the chances of the IV infiltrating.**

Note: Never cover the venipuncture site directly with tape; use a transparent dressing or sterile gauze pad first before applying tape.

1. Looping the tubing

Always loop the tubing and firmly tape the loop to the patient's skin. This helps to stabilize the catheter/needle and also brings the tubing back out of the way of the patient, attendant personnel, and visitors. IV loop devices may be attached to the end of the IV tubing to form this loop.

2. Chevron method

- Place a sterile dressing over the hub of the catheter and the insertion site. Transparent Semipermeable Membrane (TSM) dressings are preferred
- Slip a piece of ½ inch tape, sticky side up, under the hub of the catheter (or under the tubing behind the wings) and cross it over the hub (or wings) to form a chevron with the point distal to the insertion site
- Place a second piece of ½ inch tape across the hub (or wings). Be careful not to obscure the venipuncture site
- Loop the tubing and tape it to the patient with tape
- Label the dressing with the catheter gauge, date, time and your initials
- Use sufficient tape to hold the catheter firmly in place

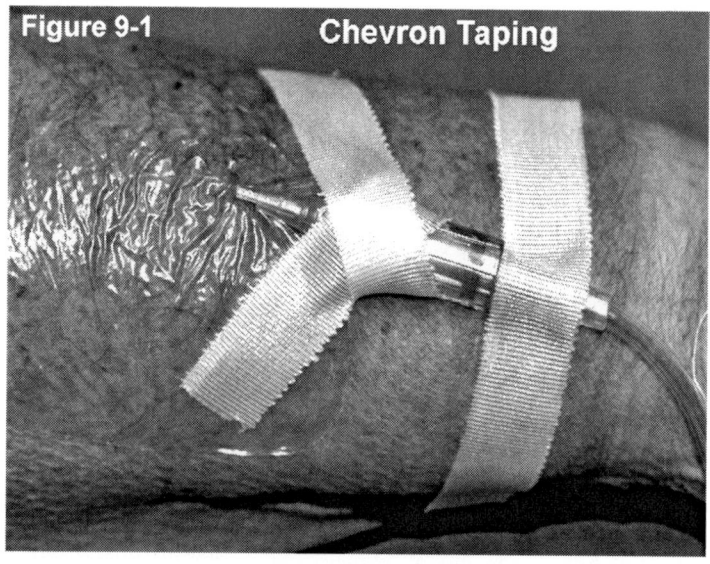

Figure 9-1   Chevron Taping

3. H method

This method of taping (Figure 9-2) may be used with winged needles.

- Place a sterile dressing over the insertion site (TSM or gauze)
- Cover each wing perpendicularly with a piece of 1-inch tape
- Cross over the wings with a piece of 1-inch tape horizontal to the first two, forming a letter H
- Loop the tubing and tape the loop to the patient with tape
- Label the dressing with the needle gauge, date, time and your initials

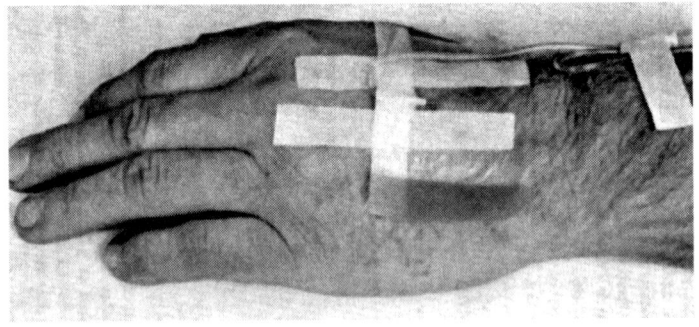

Figure 9-2. H method of taping

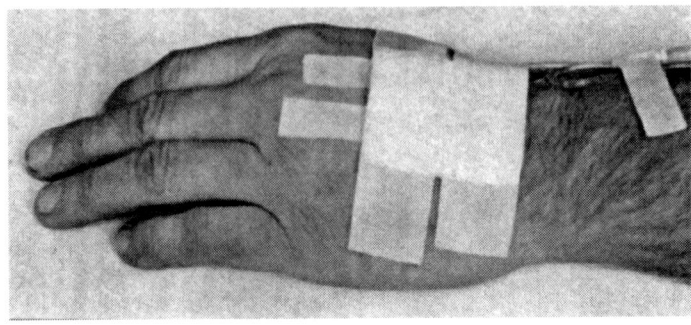

Figure 9-3. Alternative H method of taping

4. U method

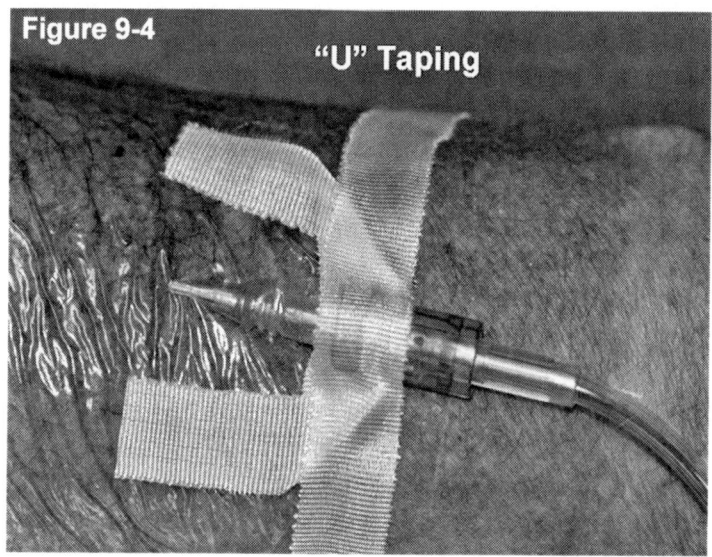

Figure 9-4   "U" Taping

This method of taping may be used with winged needles or CON devices.

- Place a sterile dressing over the insertion site (TSM or gauze)
- Slip a piece of ½ inch tape, sticky side up, under the catheter hub and fold each end over to make a "U" (parallel to the catheter or across the wings)
- Add a second piece of ½ inch tape over the catheter hub or wings
- Loop the tubing and tape the loop to the patient with tape
- Label the dressing with the needle gauge, date, time and your initials

5. Scalp-vein method

Scalp venipuncture is done primarily in infants but may occasionally be utilized in an elderly patient. You'll need to inspect the site more frequently; this method lets you do so by using a minimum of tape and protection device.

- Place a sterile dressing over the insertion site
- Tape down the wings or hub of the venipuncture device with ½ inch tape
- Make a loop in the tubing and tape the loop in place with ½-inch or 1-inch tape
- Cover the dressing with labeled ½-inch or 1-inch tape (or, if your institution permits, label the cup in the next step)
- Cut the bottom off a paper, polystyrene, or medicine cup; cut a slot in the rim; and place the cup over the dressing with the slot over the tubing
- Tape the cup to the patient's head

6. Special tips

a. *Length.* Tapes that go around the patient's extremity may be long enough to meet at the ends. Then, if the patient becomes diaphoretic, the tape will not fall off. But do not continuously wrap the tape around the patient's extremity; it then would act as a tourniquet.

b. *Backing.* If the IV is placed in an especially hairy area, back the tape with gauze or another piece of tape. Do not shave the area (see Chapter 7).

c. *More taping.* Do not hesitate to use as much tape as necessary to immobilize the catheter/needle and stabilize the tubing. For instance, it may be helpful to apply a piece of tape further up the patient's arm to help absorb tension on the line.

d. *Size.* If the IV is located in a finger, or if the patient is an infant, you may want to use smaller tape (1/4 inch instead of 1/2 inch or 1/2 inch instead of 1 inch) and use a tongue depressor to stabilize the area.

e. *Transparent dressings.*

  a. Transparent semipermeable (TSM) dressings allow for clear visualization of the venipuncture site
  b. However, you will still need to stabilize the catheter hub, or wings, of the IV device after applying the transparent dressing (e.g., Op-site, Tegaderm, Bioclusive, etc.).

f. ***Specially designed stabilizing devices*** (i.e. stat locks, etc.) are also beneficially in securing an intravenous line/device.

D. BOARDS AND RESTRAINTS

The use of stabilizing boards and restraints are only permitted as indicated by your facility's policies and procedures.

1. When to use a board

Use a board when the infusion is started in the wrist or antecubital fossa area, or when the position of the extremity is important to maintain the IV flow rate. Use a long arm board for the antecubital fossa (see Chapter 7), a short hand board for the wrist, and a tongue depressor for a finger.

2. Positioning the board

Place the patient's hand on the board, palm down with the fingers extending well over the end of the board. Tell the patient to move his/her fingers frequently to help circulation and prevent stiffness.

3. Taping the board

Tape the board both above and below the joint to be immobilized. Do not apply the tape so tightly that it restricts the flow of the IV solution. Back the tape or wrap the patient's arm with gauze where necessary.

4. Restraints

Restraining the patient or wrapping the extremity with gauze may be necessary if the patient is:

- Uncooperative
- Disoriented
- An infant
- Likely to pull the IV out

Never place a restraint over or above the IV site; it will act as a tourniquet. You may place a restraint below the IV site, or attach the restraint to a board and then tape the patient's hand to the board. Check the patient frequently for irritation and infiltration. Follow your institutions policies and procedures regarding the use of restraints.

E. ADJUSTING THE FLOW RATE

1. Calculation

The orders for administering an IV infusion usually specify the total amount of fluid in liters over the total time in hours, **or the number of ml to be given per hour,** leaving you to figure out how many drops should be infused per minute.

  a. *Formula.* The following formula may be used with any IV tubing or rate of flow:

  ➢ Divide the total amount of fluid in milliliters by the total time in minutes to get the amount per minute.
  ➢ Multiply the amount per minute by the capacity of the drip chamber (10, 15, 20, or 60 drops/ml) to get the number of drops per minute.

  To illustrate, let us apply the formula to the following example:

  The orders specify 1 liter (1,000 ml) of fluid to be given in six hours (360 minutes). The drip chamber has a capacity of 15 drops/ml.

$$\frac{1,000}{360} \times 15 = 42 \text{ drops/minute.}$$

  b. *Shortcut method.* A shortcut method may be applied when using a 10, 15, or 20 drops/ml tubing and the doctor has ordered a specific amount per hour. For example:

> The orders specify 180 ml per hour and you are using a 10 drops/ml tubing. Divide the 180 ml/hour by 6:

$$\frac{180 \text{ ml/hour}}{6} = 30 \text{ drops/minute.}$$

> The orders specify 180 ml per hour and you are using a 15 drops/ml tubing. Divide the 180 ml/hour by 4:

$$\frac{180 \text{ ml/hour}}{4} = 45 \text{ drops/minute.}$$

> The orders specify 180 ml per hour and you are using a 20 drops/ml tubing. Divide the 180 ml/hour by 3:

$$\frac{180 \text{ ml/hour}}{3} = 60 \text{ drops/minute.}$$

c. **Microdrip tubing.** When regulating microdrip tubing (60 drops/ml), there is a direct correlation between the number of milliliters ordered per hour and the number of drops per minute the drip rate is set at. For example:

> The orders specify 80 ml per hour and you are using a 60 drops/ml tubing: The IV would be set at 80 drops/minute.

d. **KVO rates.** KVO rates are usually 10 drops/minute (60 ml/hour) with a standard drip set and 20 drops/ minute (20 ml/hour) when you use a microdrip set. However, individual policies regarding KVO rates may vary from one institution to another.

2. Regulator clamp

a. **Calibrated.** Turn the dial to the desired setting.

b. **Noncalibrated.** Count the number of drops that enter the drip chamber during a one-minute period. Adjust the clamp as needed.

c. **Checking.** Check the clamp and flow rate periodically, as the clamp may slip or be tampered with.

d. **Tampering.** Warn the patient not to disturb the clamp and instruct him/her to tell visitors not to touch it.

F. LABELING AND DOCUMENTATION

Labeling and charting are just as necessary as the other steps in IV therapy. Labeling communicates information to other personnel and serves as a reminder to change tubing and dressings.

1. Labeling the bottle/bag

The following information should be on a label on the IV container (this is often on the container prepared by the pharmacy). If the information label is not provided, or you are adding a medication to an IV solution, you will need to make your own label:

- **Patient's name, and ID number**
- Name of the drug
- Dosage—the amount and period of time as ordered by the physician
- Flow rate—the number of drops per minute that you calculated
- Date and time the infusion was started
- Container number—how many containers the patient has received (if your institution requires this information)

2. Labeling the tubing

Write on a label or piece of tape the date and time the administration set was added. Then fold the label or tape around the tubing to make a tab.

3. Labeling the dressing

Write on a label or piece of 1-inch tape the size and type of venipuncture device, the date and time, and your initials. Place the label or tape on top of the dressing as described in section C above.

4. Charting

The patient's record must include the following information:

- The number of attempts made to start the line
- Type and amount of solution hung
- Size and type of venipuncture device
- Date and time
- Site of venipuncture
- Rate of infusion
- Pertinent observations, such as fainting, etc.
- Reason for discontinuation of a previous IV (e.g., hematoma, infiltration, phlebitis)
- The name of the person starting the infusion (you)

NOTE: All patient records are legal documents. Always write entries in ink. Never erase, use correction fluid, or cross something out so that it becomes illegible. If you make an error, draw a single line through the incorrect word(s) and write the word "error," the date and time, and your initials above it. Then write in the correct information (see Chapter 24).

CHAPTER 10

Midline Catheters

Patients requiring several weeks or months of IV therapy, or those with poor venous access, may require a more substantial line than that provided by the routine CON device or winged needle. The type of device chosen will depend on the type of therapy, the condition of the patient's peripheral and central venous access, the length of therapy, the patient and physician's preferences.

A. DESCRIPTION

A midline catheter does not enter the central circulatory system but provides a stable access within the peripheral circulatory system. Midline catheters are currently produced in either single or double lumen. They are generally inserted in the basilic, median cubital or cephalic veins just above or below the antecubital fossa. Midline catheters range from 3" to 8" in length and are indicated for patients with limited peripheral veins or those requiring several weeks of intravenous therapy. Midline catheters do not require a post x-ray to verify placement since they remain within the peripheral vasculature.

B. UTILIZATION

1. These catheters may be utilized for many therapies, including PPN (peripheral parenteral nutrition), some antibiotics, hydration and analgesic therapy. They should not be used for TPN (total

parenteral nutrition), vesicant drugs or for medications with a high osmolarity, requiring a large hemodilution.

2. Hemostats or clamps with teeth should not be used on these catheters due to possible damaging of the catheter.

3. Blood pressure cuffs or tourniquets should not be placed on the arm where a midline catheter is in place.

4. Midline catheters should only be **placed by nurses who have received special training/certification in the insertion process.**

C. PREPARATION FOR INSERTION:

1. Verify the physician's order for IV solution, medication (if ordered), and flow rate.
2. Check the patient's allergy history.
3. Choose the appropriate equipment:

   ➢ Midline vascular access device (choose the smallest size catheter that will meet the patient's needs).

   NOTE: Most PICC lines (see Chapter 11) may be cut for midline insertion but many manufacturers produce catheters specifically made for Midline insertion.

   ➢ Sterile insertion tray (includes: sterile drapes, 3 alcohol swabsticks, 3 povidone-iodine swabsticks, tourniquet, sterile gloves, mask, sterile scissors, sterile tape, sterile dressing)
   ➢ Flush solution & syringe (5ml of 100u heparin flush or 0.9% sodium chloride flush. If a closed-end catheter is being used only the 0.9% sodium chloride flush is necessary)
   ➢ IV solution, tubing, prn adapter & IV pole if appropriate

4. Label the IV bag/bottle if IV solution is to be infused. Inspect the solution for color, clarity, presence of particulate matter, expiration date, and general integrity of the system. Discard if defects or contamination are detected.

5. If an IV solution is to be used, attach the tubing to the fluid and prime the tubing.
6. Identify the patient.
7. Explain the procedure to the patient.
8. Remove any articles that may constrict or be in the way of starting, observing, or maintaining the line.
9. Position the patient in a supine position. Extend the patient's arm fully and support the elbow with a rolled towel or pillow as needed.
10. Provide adequate lighting and privacy.
11. Wash your hands.

D. PROCEDURE

1. Open the insertion tray and prepare a sterile field. Place a drape or chux underneath the patient's arm to protect the bed linen and patient from possible soiling from blood.
2. Apply the tourniquet and assess the condition of the veins in the antecubital area. Determine the condition of the veins by observation and palpation, checking for sclerosing, bruising, tenderness and presence of an aberrant artery. The insertion site should be just *above or below* the antecubital fossa in the basilic, median cubital or cephalic vein to insure maximum comfort and stable placement. The line should not be started directly in the antecubital area as this may impede the flow of solution or cause kinking or breaking of the catheter.
3. Don sterile gloves.
4. Cleanse the skin with the alcohol swabsticks starting from the anticipated puncture site in a circular motion out to the periphery (about 3 inches). Use a firm friction rub. Repeat this process three times using each swabstick only once.
5. Repeat the process with the three povidone-iodine swabsticks. Allow the povidone-iodine solution to dry on the patient's skin.

NOTE: Some facilities and line manufacturers are now using Chlorhexidine Gluconate (Cloraprep®) in place of the alcohol and povidone-iodine cleansing prep. Either method of preparatory cleansing is acceptable.

6. Drape the patient's arm so that the entire catheter may be placed on the drape while maintaining sterility.
7. Remove the guard from the catheter and prepare the catheter for insertion according to the manufacturer's instructions.
8. Perform the venipuncture.
9. Release the tourniquet by using a sterile 4x4 or with the drape in order to prevent contamination of your gloves. Remove the stylet and slowly advance the catheter per the manufacturer's instructions. You may want to flush the catheter with 0.9% sodium chloride solution as you advance it to help ease the insertion process.
10. Secure the catheter with a sterile dressing over the venipuncture site and stabilize with tape as needed.
11. Remove the guide wire and attach the primed IV tubing or attach the PRN adapter.
12. Tape the IV tubing/catheter to the patient's arm to help absorb tension on the line and set the infusion rate or flush the catheter with 3-5ml of 100unit heparin flush solution or 0.9% sodium chloride flush.
13. Label the IV site dressing with the date, time, size of catheter, and your initials.
14. Remove your gloves.
15. Instruct the patient to report any sensations of pain, burning, swelling, or drainage at once.
16. Properly dispose of or return equipment to the appropriate place.
17. Wash your hands.
18. Document the procedure on the patient's record.
19. Midline catheters may also be inserted utilizing Ultra Sound & Modified Seldinger technique. See Chapter 11 (PICC line insertion).

E. MAINTENANCE

1. Dressings should be changed at least once a week and prn using sterile technique (some physicians/institutions may require a more frequent dressing change).
2. These catheters may remain in place for several weeks if no complications (e.g. infiltration, phlebitis) develop that necessitate its removal. The length of time these catheters may

remain in place will vary depending on the type of material the catheter is made of, the catheter placement, the institutions policy and the manufacturers recommendations.

3. If the catheter is not used for a continuous infusion a PRN adapter should be attached to the distal end of the catheter and the catheter flushed with 3-5 ml of 100 unit heparin flush solution[ ] once a day to maintain patency of the catheter(if it is a closed-end or valved catheter—then only 0.9% NSS needs to be used to flush the line.)

[ ]   To maintain the patency of various IV catheters, some institutions are using 10 ml heparin flush solution and some are simply using 0.9 NSS instead. The type of flush solution utilized does not appear to be significant in maintaining catheter patency in most instances. Whichever solution your institution requires is all right, as long as it sufficiently maintains the patency of the catheter.

CHAPTER 11

Central Line Catheters

Patients requiring several months or years of IV therapy will require a stable route of delivery that is best accommodated by the insertion of a central line. The type of central line utilized will be determined by the condition of the patient's peripheral and central venous systems, the length and type of therapy, and the patient and physicians preferences.

A. *PICC LINES* (Peripherally inserted central catheters)

1. Description

A peripherally inserted central catheter is generally inserted by a physician or specially trained RN (state regulations vary regarding who may perform this procedure and under what conditions). A PICC line is generally inserted in the basilic, median cubital or cephalic veins just above or below the antecubital fossa. PICC lines are currently available in single, double and triple lumen. There are also "power" PICC lines which may be used by Diagnostic Imaging for power injections. The distal tip of the catheter is generally threaded into the superior vena cava. Once the catheter has been inserted, placement must be confirmed by chest x-ray prior to initiation of therapy.

2. Utilization

- PICC lines may be utilized for all types of IV therapies including TPN, chemotherapy, antibiotics and analgesics.
- Hemostats or clamps with teeth should not be used on these catheters due to possible damaging of the catheter.
- Blood pressure cuffs or tourniquets should not be placed on the arm where a PICC line is in place.
- PICC lines may only be inserted by physicians or nurses who have received special training/certification in the procedure.
- PICC lines are contraindicated for:

  o patients with lack of peripheral venous access (these patients may need to be referred to interventional radiology to have a PICC inserted under fluoroscopy).
  o venous thrombosis (these patients may need to be referred to interventional radiology to have a PICC inserted under fluoroscopy).
  o chronic renal failure or end-stage renal disease (the need to preserve peripheral veins for future dialysis fistulas is critical for these patients).

3. Preparation for insertion

- Verify the physicians order for IV solution, medication (if ordered) and flow rate
- A consent form should be signed by the patient
- Check the patient's allergy history
- Choose the appropriate equipment

NOTE: There are several types of PICC lines on the market

a. PICC line
b. Flush solution & syringe with 3-5ml of 100 unit heparin flush solution and 10ml 0.9% normal saline solution for flushing
c. IV solution, tubing & pole or PRN adapter & ext. tubing
d. Vial of 0.9 saline solution

e. Sterile gloves (2 pair)
f. Mask
g. Sterile drapes
h. 1% Lidocaine (3-5ml)

NOTE: Many sterile insertion trays come with all the necessary supplies. Some have the PICC catheter in the tray and for others you may need to add the appropriate PICC catheter.

- Label the IV bag/bottle, if an IV solution is to be infused. Inspect the solution for color, clarity, presence of particulate matter, expiration date and general integrity of the system. Discard if defects or contamination are detected.
- If an IV solution is to be used, attach the tubing to the fluid and prime the tubing.
- Identify the patient.
- Explain the procedure to the patient.
- Remove any articles of clothing that may constrict or be in the way of starting, observing or maintaining the line.
- Position the patient in a supine position. The patient's arm should be abducted from the patient's body. Extend the arm fully and support the elbow with a rolled towel, pillow or sheet as needed.
- Provide adequate lighting and privacy.
- Wash your hands.

4. Procedure for direct insertion with peel-away cannula technique:

- Using the clean measuring tape, measure the distance from the anticipated insertion site up the arm and across the clavicle to the suprasternal notch then down 3 intercostal spaces (3-inches) for superior vena cava placement; add an additional 1-2 inches for the external portion of the catheter.
- Apply the tourniquet to the patient's arm and assess the veins in the antecubital fossa. Determine the condition of the veins by observation and palpation, checking for sclerosing, bruising, tenderness and presence of an aberrant artery. The insertion site should be just above or below the antecubital fossa in the

basilic vein, the median cubital vein or the cephalic vein. This location will insure maximum comfort and stable placement.

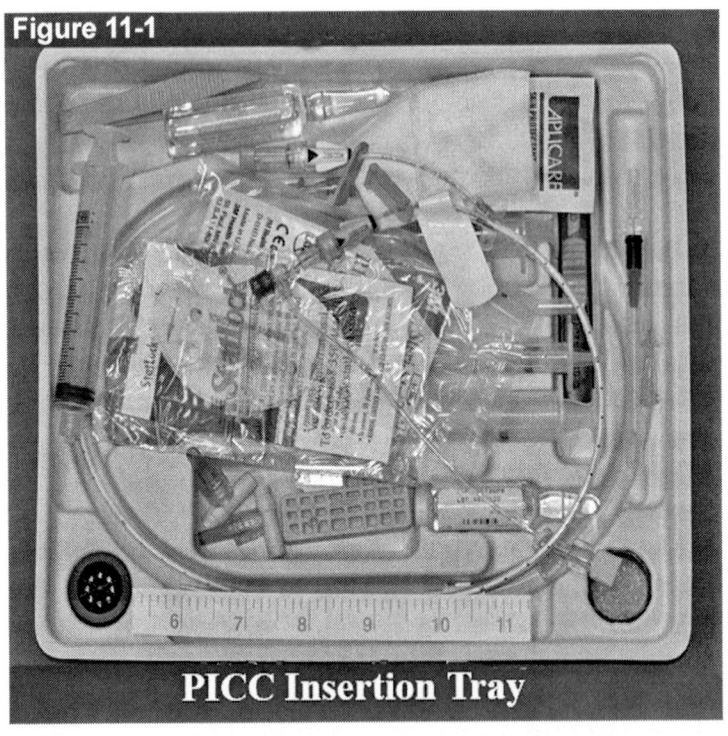

Figure 11-1

PICC Insertion Tray

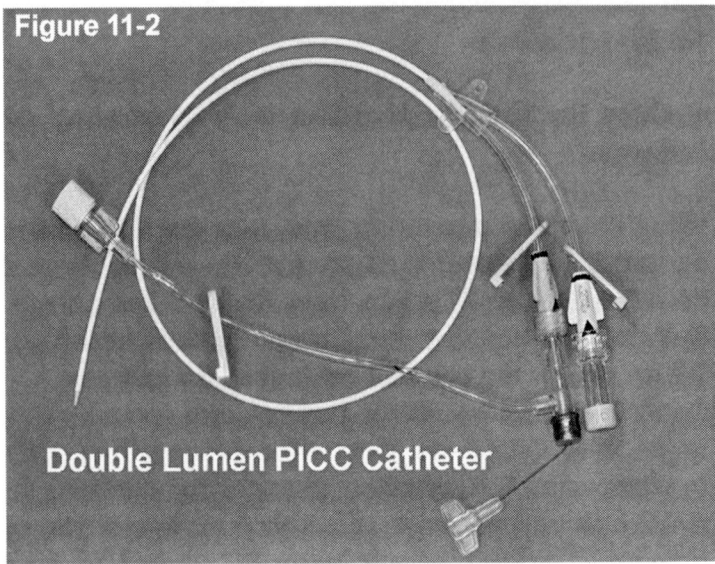

Figure 11-2

Double Lumen PICC Catheter

- Remove the tourniquet but leave it under the patient's arm
- Don the mask
- Open sterile insertion tray and prepare sterile field
- Add to the tray, using sterile technique, any additional equipment required
- Don sterile gloves
- Place the moisture proof pad under the patient's arm
- Cleanse the skin with the alcohol swabsticks starting from the anticipated puncture site in a circular motion out to the periphery (about 3-inches). Use a firm friction rub. Repeat this process three times using each swabstick only once.
- Repeat the cleansing procedure with the povidone-iodine swabsticks.

NOTE: Some facilities and line manufacturers are now using Chlorhexidine Gluconate (Cloraprep®) in place of the alcohol and povidone-iodine cleansing prep. Either method of preparatory cleansing is acceptable.

- Inject (intradermally) 0.5 to 1 ml of 1% Lidocaine, at the intended site.
- Remove the guidewire from the catheter (the guidewire may be left in place if you prefer and your state allows the use of a guidewire).
- Using the sterile measuring tape, measure the catheter to the desired length and cut the distal end to the pre-measured length.

It is preferable to cut the catheter straight across and not at an angle. If you are using a closed-end (Groshong) catheter the proximal end will be cut and **NOT** the distal end. (If the guidewire is to be used, pull the guidewire back to the pre-measured length and bend the wire at the proximal end prior to cutting the distal end.)

- Using sterile technique, withdraw 5-10ml of 0.9 NSS from the vial and flush the PRN cap & extension tubing. Then remove the syringe and flush the catheter with 0.9 NSS to assure

patency and to make the catheter more firm for threading;
leave the syringe in place. It is not necessary to flush the
catheter if a guidewire is to be used.

- Apply the tourniquet and remove the contaminated gloves
- With the second pair of sterile gloves, drape the patient's
  arm with the sterile drape
- Place a sterile gauze over the tourniquet
- Remove the guard from the introducer needle and perform
  the venipuncture through the lidocaine wheal
- When blood return is obtained, advance the catheter through
  the needle, approximately 2-3 inches into the vein
- Using the sterile gauze, release the tourniquet
- Continue to advance the catheter through the introducer
  needle with the tweezers until approximately 6-8 inches
  have been threaded
- Gently withdraw the introducer needle out of the patient's
  skin. Hold the catheter with the tweezers at the distal end
  and slide the needle towards the hub of the catheter.
- Squeeze the wings of the needle together and peel away the
  needle (or remove the needle according to the manufacturers
  instructions)

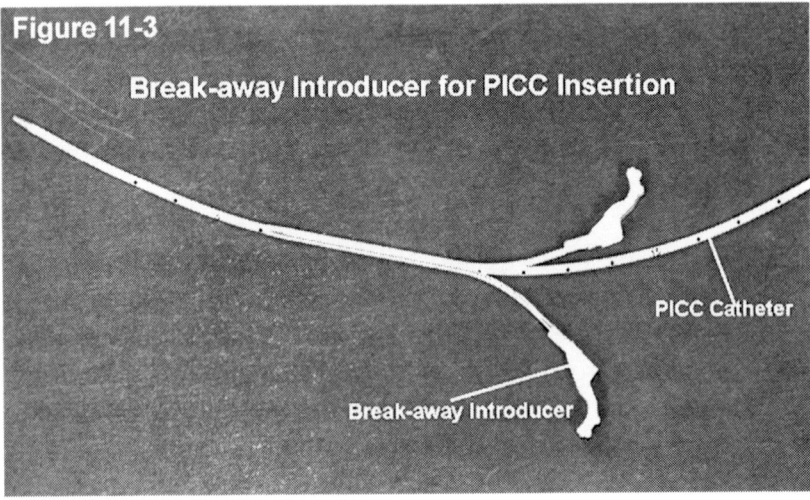

Figure 11-3

Break-away Introducer for PICC Insertion

PICC Catheter

Break-away Introducer

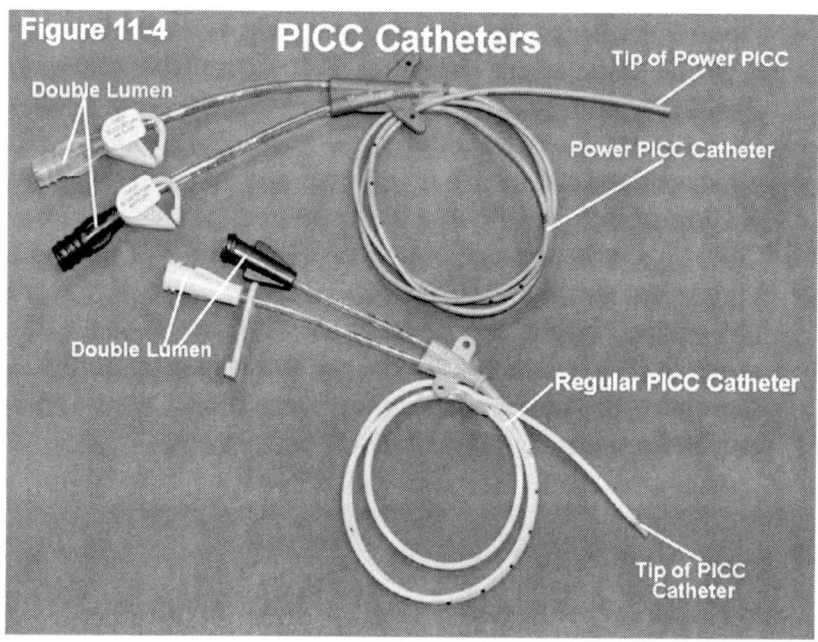

Figure 11-4 — **PICC Catheters**

- Have the patient turn his/her head towards the insertion arm and place their chin on the shoulder near the clavicle. Have them hold this position until the pre-measured length of catheter has been inserted (there should be approximately 2-inches remaining). This will help occlude the jugular vein and facilitate the catheter advancement into the superior vena cava.
- Continue to advance the catheter according to your initial measurements for proper catheter tip placement. (If a guidewire is used, remove the guidewire and attach the syringe with the 0.9 NSS.)
- Aspirate for a blood return and then flush the catheter with 10ml 0.9% NSS.
- Remove the syringe and apply the extension set with the PRN adapter to the hub of the catheter.
- Leave a little slack in the catheter to help absorb tension, and secure the catheter with one or two sutures, a catheter securing device or steri-strips.

- Place a sterile gauze over the insertion site and then apply a sterile transparent dressing. This should be removed in 24-48 hrs. and a new transparent (TSM) dressing applied.
- Remove the gloves and tape the extension tubing in place.
- Flush catheter with 3-5 ml of 100 unit heparin. Flush with 5-10ml of 0.9%NS if using a closed end or valved catheter.
- Obtain a chest x-ray for verification of tip placement. Placement should be in the superior vena cava. If placement is verified, begin the prescribed therapy: if the catheter needs to be pulled back, remove the dressing, gently slide the catheter out the appropriate length and apply another sterile dressing. Re-xray to verify placement.

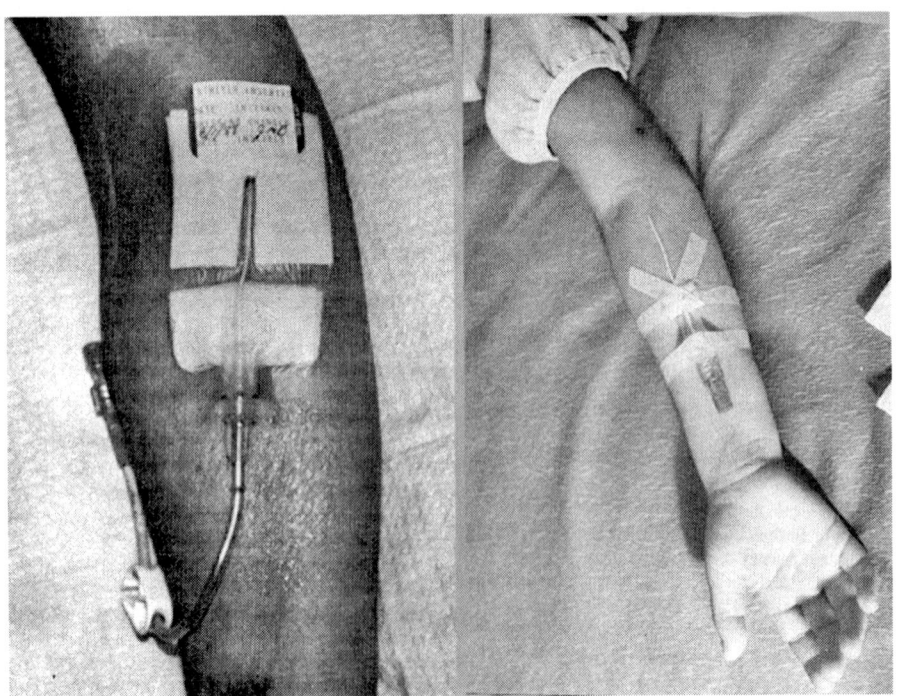

Figure 11-5. Insertion site of an adult   **Figure 11-6.** Insertion site of a child

- Instruct the patient not to pull on the catheter and to report any sensations of pain, burning, swelling or drainage at once.
- Properly dispose of or return equipment to the appropriate place.
- Wash your hands.

- Document the procedure on the patient's chart: include the length of catheter inserted, tip placement, how the patient tolerated the procedure and any difficulties encountered.

5. Ultrasound and Modified Seldinger Technique

- An Ultrasound machine is utilized to view the peripheral veins and help determine appropriate placement. Ultrasound also facilitates the access of larger veins in the upper arm which are more desirable for PICC placement.
- Preparation for insertion (same as #3 above)
- Use the measuring tape and measure the distance from the anticipated insertion site up the arm and across the clavicle to the suprasternal notch then down 3 intercostal spaces (3-inches) for superior vena cava placement; add an additional 1-2 inches for the external portion of the catheter.
- Apply the tourniquet and remove the contaminated gloves
- Locate the best vein for inserting the PICC utilizing the Ultra Sound
- The insertion site should be just above or below the antecubital fossa in the basilic vein, the median cubital vein or the cephalic vein. Veins accessed in the upper arm have been associated with a lower incidence of thrombosis, phlebitis and catheter migration.
- Don the mask
- Open sterile insertion tray and prepare sterile field
- Add to the tray, using sterile technique, any additional equipment required
- Don sterile gloves
- Place the moisture proof pad under the patient's arm
- Cleanse the skin with the alcohol swabsticks starting from the anticipated puncture site in a circular motion out to the periphery (about 3-inches). Use a firm friction rub. Repeat this process three times using each swabstick only once. Repeat the cleansing procedure with the povidone-iodine swabsticks.

NOTE: Some facilities and line manufacturers are now using Chlorhexidine Gluconate (Cloraprep®) in place of the alcohol and povidone-iodine cleansing prep. Either method of preparatory cleansing is acceptable.

- Inject (intradermally) 0.5-1 ml of 1% Lidocaine, at the intended insertion site.
- Access the vein, through the lidocaine wheal, with the intravenous cannula or needle provided in the PICC line tray.
- A guide wire is threaded into the needle or cannula approximately 4-6 inches then the needle or cannula is removed, leaving the guide wire in place.
- A small nick is made with the scalpel in the skin beside the guide wire, and the introducer sheath with dilator is inserted over the guide wire.
- The guide wire and dilator are removed and the catheter is advanced through the introducer sheath, approximately 4 inches.
- Remove the tourniquet with a gauze pad to maintain sterility of your gloves.
- The catheter is advanced to the designated length and then the introducer sheath is pulled back and peeled away after the catheter has been threaded.
- Leave a little slack in the catheter to help absorb tension, and secure the catheter with one or two sutures, a catheter securing device or steri-strips.
- Place a sterile gauze over the insertion site and then apply a sterile transparent dressing. This should be removed in 24-48 hrs. and a new transparent (TSM) dressing applied.
- Remove the gloves and tape the extension tubing in place.
- Flush the catheter with 10ml 0.9% NSS
- Flush catheter with 3-5 ml of 100 unit heparin/saline flush.
- Obtain a chest x-ray for verification of tip placement. Placement should be in the superior vena cava. If placement is verified, begin the prescribed therapy: if the catheter needs to be pulled back, remove the dressing, gently slide

the catheter out the appropriate length and apply another sterile dressing. Re-xray to verify placement.

- Instruct the patient not to pull on the catheter and to report any sensations of pain, burning, swelling or drainage at once.
- Properly dispose of or return equipment to the appropriate place.
- Wash your hands.
- Document the procedure on the patient's chart: include the length of catheter inserted, tip placement, how the patient tolerated the procedure and any difficulties encountered.

6. Maintenance

- Dressings should be changed within the first 24-48hrs. to remove the gauze dressing. Then a sterile transparent dressing should be applied to the site and changed at least once a week and prn using sterile technique. A *Biopatch* (impregnated with chlorhexidine Gluconate) may be applied. The *Biopatch* provides antimicrobial action for up to 7 days.
- These catheters may remain in place for up to one year if no complications (e.g. phlebitis) develop that necessitate its removal (consult the manufacturers recommendations for the length of time the catheter may be left in place).
- If the catheter is not used for a continuous infusion a PRN adapter should be attached to the distal end of the catheter.
- PRN adapters and/or extension tubings should be changed once a week and prn.

7. Potential complications:

- Injury to tissues, arteries, nerves, or tendons at the insertion site can be prevented by choosing palpable, resilient veins that can be entered without probing. Utilizing the Ultrasound to locate an acceptable vein will decrease the need to "probe".
- ***Phlebitis***—Assess the site daily for pain, warmth, erythema or edema. Apply warm, moist compresses without removing

the catheter and notify the physician. If the phlebitis resolves within 24-48 hrs., the catheter may not need to be removed. The phlebitis may be due to mechanical or chemical irritation. If the phlebitis persists over 48hrs. the PICC may need to be removed and a culture done on the catheter/site.

- **Thrombosis**—Check the area for swelling around the shoulder, neck and/or face, shoulder stiffness, or difficulty aspirating blood. Notify the physician. A radiological examination may be indicated; if confirmed, anti-coagulant therapy may be ordered.
- **Air Embolus**—This may be prevented by maintaining the level of the insertion site below the heart during tubing, extension set or prn adapter changes.
- **Infection**—Check the insertion site daily for any signs of pain, edema, erythema or exudate. Notify the physician if present. A culture may be ordered.
- **Catheter slippage**—If catheter slippage is detected, do **NOT** attempt to push the catheter back into the patient's arm. Notify the physician. An x-ray may be necessary to confirm placement and/or appropriate continuation of the therapy.
- Catheter Occlusion—Most PICC line occlusions can be cleared:

  ➤ Thrombotic occlusions may be cleared with low-dose alteplase
  ➤ Lipid occlusions may be cleared with 70% ethyl alcohol
  ➤ Crystllized medications with a high pH may be cleared with sodium bicarbonate
  ➤ Crystilized medications with a low pH may be cleared with hydrochloric acid

8. Removing the catheter

- Don gloves
- Carefully remove the dressing
- Lightly cover the insertion site with a sterile gauze pad

- Grasp the exposed catheter with your gloved hand and with a smooth steady motion gently pull the catheter out 3-4 inches. Grasp the catheter again at the exit site and pull out another 3-4 inches. Continue this process until the catheter is completely removed.
- Apply digital pressure to the site with the sterile gauze pad until the bleeding stops. Then cover the site with gauze and tape and tell the patient to keep the site covered for 24 hrs.
- Check the tip of the catheter to see if it is intact.
- Measure the length of the catheter removed and compare it with the insertion length recorded in the patient's medical chart. Any discrepancy must be reported to the physician immediately and the patient kept supine and quiet.
- Properly dispose of or return equipment to the appropriate place.
- Remove gloves.
- Wash your hands.
- Record the procedure in the patient's record.

B. PLAIN CENTRAL LINES

1. Description

A plain central venous catheter (CVC) is generally inserted in the subclavian or jugular vein with the tip located in the superior vena cava. However, they may also be inserted in the femoral veins. Plain central lines are currently available in single, double, triple and quad lumens. They are frequently referred to as TLC (triple lumen catheter) or non-tunneled percutaneously inserted CVC.

2. Utilization

- These catheters are generally inserted on patients requiring several weeks (1-4 weeks) of multiple therapies where a long term catheter is not desired and/or the patient has poor peripheral venous access. These catheters may be utilized on a continuous or intermittent basis, or both.

- Plain central lines may be used for all types of therapies including TPN, chemotherapy, antibiotics and analgesics.
- Whenever connecting or disconnecting these lines it is important to clamp them to prevent excessive bleeding or the possibility of an air embolism.

3. Preparation for insertion

These catheters are generally inserted in the emergency room, the patient's hospital room or the operating room by the physician.

4. Approaching the patient

Explain the procedure to the patient and try to answer any questions or concerns he/she may have about the procedure.

5. Dressing

- The venipuncture site must be kept clean and dry at all times
- Clean the area with alcohol swabs from the center of the site to the periphery
- Clean the area with povidone-iodine swabs from the center of the site to the periphery

    NOTE: Some manufacturers are now using Chlorhexidine Gluconate (Cloraprep®) in their central line dressing change kits in place of the alcohol and povidone-iodine swabs. Either method of cleansing the central line site is acceptable.

- You may choose to place a protective barrier solution to the skin area around the dressing site where the tape or transparent dressing will be applied.
- Allow the protective dressing solution to dry.
- Apply the transparent dressing or gauze dressing to the site—be sure all edges are secured to form an occlusive dressing. Transparent dressing are generally changed once a week and prn while gauze dressing needs to be changed at least three times a week (i.e. M-W-F) and prn. (the frequency of dressing changes may vary with the individual physician/institution).

- Loop the tubing and secure it with tape
- Label the dressing with the date
- Dispose of all equipment appropriately
- Remove gloves and wash your hands
- Chart the procedure and any pertinent observations in the patient's record. Note the following information:

  o Size of catheter, date and time it was inserted, by whom, vein used, and type of solution started
  o Instructions given to patient
  o Patient's reaction to the procedure
  o Any difficulties encountered

6. Complications

Complications occur more frequently with plain central line placements than with peripheral line insertions or other types of central lines. These complications may include:

- Pneumothorax
- Hemothorax
- Air embolism
- Thoracic duct injury
- Infection
- Hematoma
- Catheter embolism
- Brachial plexus injury

Patients should be observed closely during and immediately following line placement for signs and symptoms of possible complications.

C. OPEN-END TUNNELED CATHETERS (HICKMAN, BROVIAC, TENCKHOFF, ETC.)

1. Description

A open-end tunneled catheter is a long term, indwelling catheter, usually inserted into the superior vena cava via the subclavian vein.

The distal end of the catheter is tunneled subcutaneously over the chest wall and usually exits at the chest line. A dacron cuff around the catheter, placed approximately 2 cm subcutaneously, proximal to the exit site, allows for sclerosis of tissue in the subcutaneous tunnel forming a microbial barrier against the migration of bacteria up the skin tract. These catheters are currently available in single, double and triple lumen.

2. Utilization

These catheters may be utilized for all types of IV therapies including TPN, chemotherapy, antibiotics and analgesics.

3. Preparation for insertion

Open-end tunneled catheters are inserted by a physician in the operating room of a hospital. This may be done on an out-patient basis. Placement is verified by x-ray prior to initiation of therapy.

4. Maintenance

- If the catheter is used for intermittent therapy a PRN adapter should be placed on the distal end of the catheter.
- Hemostats or clamps with teeth should not be used on these catheters due to possible damaging of the catheter. Clamps attached to the catheter by the manufacturer should be kept closed when IV's are not being infused. The catheter should also be clamped when connecting or disconnecting IV tubings or prn adapters. Clamping is important to prevent excessive bleeding or possible air embolism.
- Dressings should be changed once a week and prn using sterile technique.
- These catheters may remain in place for several months or years if no complications (e.g. infection, venous thrombosis) develop that necessitate its removal.
- If the catheter is inadvertently pulled out, cover the exit site with a sterile gauze pad and notify the physician.

D. CLOSED-END (OR PASSIVE VALVE) TUNNELED CATHETER (EG. GROSHONG, VAXCEL, ETC.)

1. Description

A closed-end or valved tunneled catheter is a long term, indwelling catheter usually inserted into the superior vena cava via the subclavian vein. The distal end of the catheter is tunneled subcutaneously over the chest wall and usually exits at the chest line. A dacron cuff around the catheter, placed approximately 2 cm subcutaneously, proximal to the exit site, allows for sclerosis of tissue in the subcutaneous tunnel forming a microbial barrier against the migration of bacteria up the skin tract. Some of these catheters are currently available in single, and double lumen and a few are available in triple lumen.

2. Utilization

Closed-end catheters may be utilized for all types of IV therapies including TPN, chemotherapy, antibiotics and analgesics.

3. Preparation for insertion

Closed-end tunneled catheters are inserted by a physician in the operating room of a hospital. This may be done on an out-patient basis. Placement is verified by x-ray prior to initiation of therapy.

4. Maintenance

- If the catheter is used for intermittent therapy a PRN adapter should be placed on the distal end and the catheter.
- Hemostats or clamps should NOT be used on these catheters due to possible damaging of the catheter. Because of the specially designed valve system in these catheters the patient will not loose blood or inhale air when the catheter is uncapped.

- Dressings should be changed once a week and prn using sterile technique.
- These catheters may remain in place for several months or years if no complications (e.g. infection, venous thrombosis) develop that necessitate its removal.
- If the catheter is inadvertently pulled out, cover the exit site with a sterile gauze pad and notify the physician.

E. SUBCUTANEOUS PORTS (PORT-A-CATH, MEDI-PORT, INFUSA-PORT, LIFE-PORT, PASS-PORT, ETC.)

1. Description

The subcutaneous implanted central line port is a long term indwelling catheter. It is a small reservoir with a silicone center located at the distal end of the catheter. The proximal tip of the catheter is generally inserted into the superior vena cava via the subclavian vein. The distal port is generally placed under the skin in the chest area but may be located in other areas depending on physician preference. Ports are currently available in single and double lumen.

2. Utilization

Subcutaneous ports may be utilized for all types of IV therapies including TPN, chemotherapy, antibiotics and analgesics.

3. Preparation for insertion

These catheters are inserted by a physician in the operating room of a hospital. This may be done on an out-patient basis. Placement is verified by x-ray prior to initiation of therapy.

4. Maintenance

- To prevent coring of the silicone septum on the port, only special "non-coring" needles are to be used. Standard needles are never used on subcutaneous ports due to the possibility of "coring" the septum. You will know that the silicone center has been "cored" if you access the port and while fluid is infusing the area around the site and dressing will be getting wet from the IV solution.

- Dressings should be changed once a week until the insertion site is healed (some physicians/institutions require more frequent dressing changes). Once the site is healed, no dressing at the insertion site is required.
- Ports may be used for continuous or intermittent therapy.

    a. ***Accessing the Port***—don gloves and mask, cleanse the area with an 3 alcohol swabs then cleanse the area with three povidone-iodine swabs (Some facilities are now using Chlorhexidine Gluconate (Cloraprep®) in their central line dressing change kits in place of the alcohol and povidone-iodine swabs. Either method of cleansing the site is acceptable). Hold the port with one hand and the "non-coring" needle with the other hand; insert the needle into the center of the port, according to the manufacturers directions. Insert the needle completely through the silicone diaphragm until you feel the needle hit the metal at the back of the port.

    b. ***For continuous therapy***—attach the tubing attached to the "non-coring" needle to the primed IV fluid tubing then cover the site and needle with a sterile transparent dressing. Set the fluid at the designated rate of flow. Change the dressing and the needle once a week (some physicians/facilities require the dressing to be changed more frequently).

    c. ***For intermittent therapy (received more than once a day)***—access the port with the "non-coring" needle. Place a PRN adapter at the distal end of the tubing and cover the site and needle with a sterile transparent dressing. The port should be flushed with 10ml of 0.9% NSS flush solution after each infusion. The needle and the dressing should be changed once a week (some physicians/facilities require the dressing to be changed more frequently).

d. For intermittent therapy (received once a day, weekly or monthly). Access the PORT with the "non-coring" needle. Infuse the prescribed fluid/medication; flush the port with 10ml of 0.9% NSS flush then flush with 5ml of 100 units heparin flush solution; remove the needle from the port.

e. If the port in not being used and only needs to be maintained, a monthly flushing with 10ml of 0.9NSS followed with 5ml of 100 units heparin flush solution is sufficient.

- These ports may remain in place for several months or years if no complications (e.g. infection, venous thrombosis, coring of the silicone center) occur that necessitate its removal.

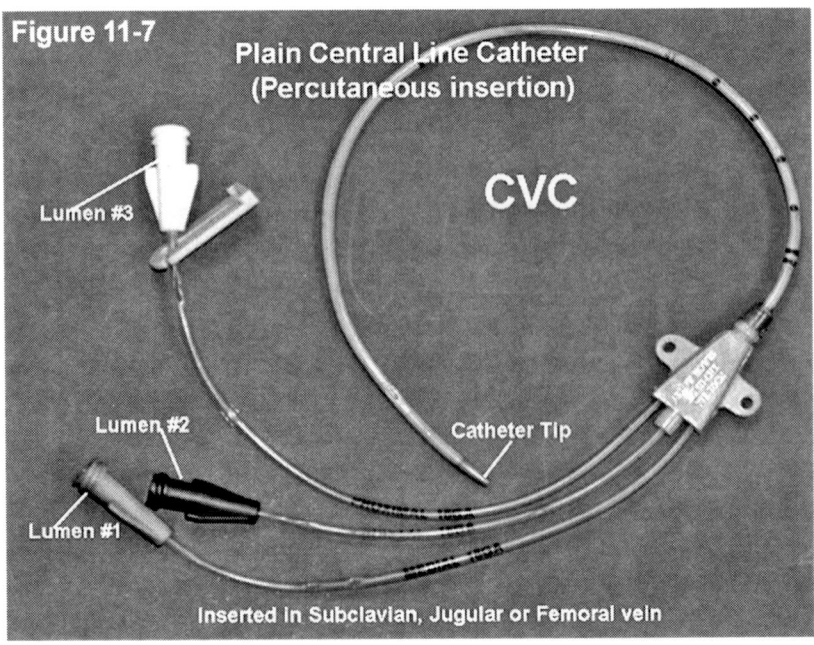

Figure 11-7 Plain Central Line Catheter (Percutaneous insertion)

CVC

Lumen #3

Lumen #2   Catheter Tip

Lumen #1

Inserted in Subclavian, Jugular or Femoral vein

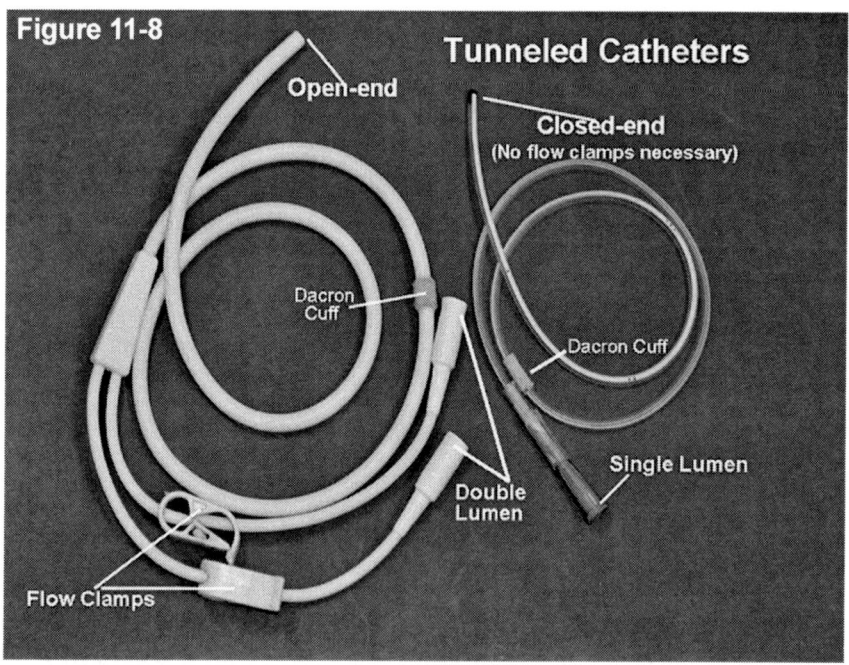

Figure 11-8 — Tunneled Catheters

5. Complications

Complications may occur with any central line placement. The most frequent reason these catheters are removed is due to infection. Complications may include:

- Infection (most frequent)
- Air embolism
- Hematoma
- Infiltration
- Formation of fibrin sheath

Patients should be observed closely for possible signs and symptoms of central line complications.

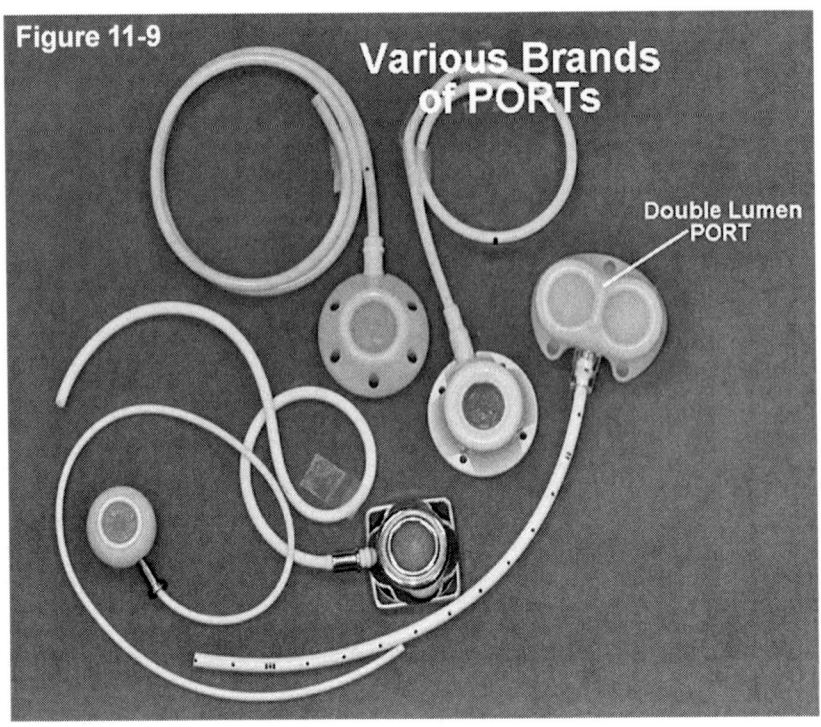

Figure 11-9

Various Brands of PORTs

Double Lumen PORT

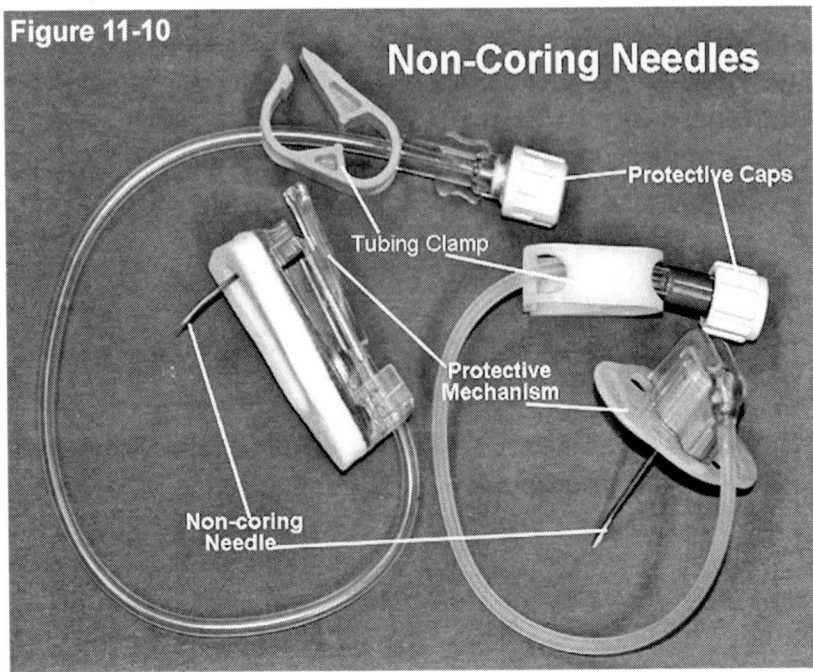

Figure 11-10

Non-Coring Needles

Protective Caps

Tubing Clamp

Protective Mechanism

Non-coring Needle

F. FLUSHING CENTRAL LINES

1. If one or more of the catheters lumens are not used for a continuous infusion, they should have a PRN adapter at the distal end of the lumen. The unused or intermittent lumens should be flushed according to you facilities policy to maintain patency of the lumen.
2. Some guidelines for consideration:

   a. Flush all central lines with 10ml 0.9% NSS solution after each infusion.
   b. Flush all closed-end/valved lines with 10ml 0.9% NSS once each infusion and/or once a week and prn when not in use.
   c. Flush all open-end catheters with Neutral or Positive Pressure prn adapter caps with 10ml 0.9% NSS after each infusion and/or once a week & prn when not in use.
   c. Flush all open-end catheters with Negative Pressure prn adapter caps with 10ml 0.9% NSS after each infusion. If used only once a day or less, flush with 10ml 0.9% NSS flush then 3-5ml of 100 units/ml heparin flush.

   (**Note:** flushing frequency, amount & strength of heparin may vary depending on physician order &/or your facility policy.)

3. Flush all central lines with 10ml of 0.9% NSS after blood is drawn.
4. Pediatric/NICU patients: 10units/ml heparin flush may be substituted for the 100units/ml flush.
5. Flush the line with 0.9% NSS before and after administration of medications.
6. Use a 10ml syringe, or greater, for flushing/injecting into a central line.

G. POWER LINES

1. Many central lines are now manufactured as "power lines".
2. Power lines are central line catheters that will withstand the "power injections" delivered by Diagnostic Imaging when doing a CAT scan.
3. Some of the manufacturers have color coded theses lines "purple"—they are known as "Purple Power Lines".
4. Prior to sending a patient to Diagnostic Imaging for a CAT scan, check to see if the patient has a "power line" (this includes power PORTs).
5. Maintenance (dressings & flushing) for power lines are the same as they are for the regular, "non-power" lines.

H. PRN ADAPTERS

Needless prn adapters allow access to IV lines which do not require the use of needles. These systems are the preferred method for accessing IV systems and very effective in helping to reduce accidental needle stick injuries. They may be used as saline or heparin locks which permit intermittent infusions.

1. PRN adapters come in Negative, Positive and Neutral designs.

   a. Positive adapters exert a slight push of force when the syringe is detached. If you need to clamp the catheter do it **after** you detach the syringe.
   b. Negative adapters exert a slight pull of force when the syringe is detached—it is important to clamp the central line **before** you detach the syringe to prevent blood from backing up into the catheter.
   c. Neutral adapters do not exert any pull or push pressure on the flush solution. If you need to clamp the catheter you may do it either before or after the flush (either way if fine).

2. PRN adapters are one of the most common sites for contamination in an IV system. The PRN adapter must be

firmly cleansed with an alcohol wipe for 10-15 seconds prior to accessing the line for *ANY* reason!

3. PRN adapter should be changed at least once a week and prn or according to you institutes policy.

I. DRAWING BLOOD FROM A CENTRAL LINE CATHETER

Blood samples may be drawn from any central line catheter. However, in approximately 25% of the central line catheters placed you will be unable to aspirate blood, due to various reasons, even though placement is accurate and confirmed by x-ray. It is perfectly safe to continue to use these catheters for IV infusions once placement is confirmed by x-ray. Sometimes you can restore the aspiration of blood by treating the catheter with a low-dose thrombolytic, Alteplase (see J below). This is especially true if the catheter is slightly occluded by blood or a fibrin flap has formed.

When drawing blood samples from central line catheters it is important to remember to withdraw a minimum of 5ml of blood and discard it before drawing the blood for the ordered tests. The saline or heparin solution in the catheter would produce inaccurate test results if it was not withdrawn and discarded first. If drawing blood from a multi-lumen catheter the infusion(s) being administered through the other lumen(s) must be stopped for 2 minutes prior to drawing the blood sample.

After drawing the blood, flush with 10ml of 0.9NSS then flush according to your established protocol/policy to maintain patency of the catheter. Restart any infusion(s) that were stopped for purposes of the blood draw.

J. USE OF ALTEPLASE FOR CENTRAL LINE CLEARANCE (CATHFLO ACTIVASE BY GENENTECH)

Alteplase, or tissue plasminogen activator (tPA), is a thrombolytic agent used to dissolve clotted blood obstructing central venous access devices, fibrin sheaths or fibrin flaps. Catheters may be occluded by substances other than blood, such as precipitates.

Alteplase is not effective in those circumstances and should not be attempted.

1. Obtain an order from the physician for two vials of Alteplase (you may need to use two injections—so have a spare on hand).
2. Obtain two vials of Alteplase from the pharmacy.
3. Explain the procedure to the patient. Include the purpose and how to exhale and hold your breathe during IV tubing/syringe changes (or use a clamp on the tubing if available) to prevent air from entering the central venous system.
4. Aseptically disconnect IV tubing at the connection of the catheter hub and attach an empty 10ml syringe. Attempt to aspirate clotted material from the catheter with gentle pressure. This step must proceed the use of tPA. If aspiration is not possible, proceed to next step.

   a. Reconstitute the Alteplase per manufacturers instructions (2mg/2ml)
   b. Reconstitute immediately before use
   c. Discard reconstituted medication if not used within 8 hrs.

5. **Treating a partial thrombotic occlusion of a central venous access.**

   a. Attach the Alteplase-filled syringe to the external hub of the catheter.
   b. Unclamp the catheter and slowly instill the Alteplase solution to fill the lumen.
   c. Re-clamp the catheter, remove the syringe, and aseptically cap the hub.
   d. Proceed to no.7 below.

6. **Treating a total thrombotic occlusion of a central venous catheter**

   a. Attach a three-way stopcock to the catheter hub.

b. Attach the Alteplase-filled syringe to the stopcock port opposite the catheter hub and an empty 10ml syringe to the side port.

c. Turn off the stopcock to the Alteplase-filled syringe which will open the stopcock to the empty syringe.

d. Pull back on the empty syringe plunger to the 8ml mark, and while maintaining pressure, turn off the stopcock to the empty syringe which will open the stopcock to the Alteplase-filled syringe.

e. Allow the Alteplase solution to slowly fill the lumen.

f. Re-clamp the catheter, remove the stopcock, and aseptically cap the hub.

g. Proceed to no.7 below.

7. After 30min. of dwell time clamp the catheter and remove the cap.

a. Attach an empty 10ml syringe to the external hub of the catheter, unclamp the catheter, and attempt to aspirate 5ml of fluid/blood—continue the attempt to aspirate fluid/blood until successful every 30 min. for up to 2 hours.

   i. *If able to aspirate fluid*, clamp the catheter, discard the solution, and attach a syringe filled with 0.9% sodium chloride. Unclamp and flush the catheter with 20 ml of NSS.

   ii. *If unable to aspirate*, after 2 hours, instill a second dose of Alteplase as described above. Repeat steps 6 above. If the catheter remains occluded after 2 doses of Alteplase, contact the physician to consider alternate etiologies, potential diagnostic approaches, and additional management strategies.

8. Lipid occlusions may be cleared with 70% ethyl alcohol.

9. Crystllized medications with a high pH may be cleared with sodium bicarbonate.

10. Crystilized medications with a low pH may be cleared with hydrochloric acid.

K. IMPLANTABLE PUMPS (EG. INFUSAID)

1. Description

The implantable pump is a long term indwelling catheter with a large (approximately 50ml) reservoir at the distal end. The proximal tip of the catheter is generally inserted into the epidural or intrathecal space or directly into an organ (i.e. liver) The distal port is usually placed in the lower right or left quadrant.

2. Utilization

These pumps are used for:

- management of severe pain by placing the proximal end into the epidural or intrathecal space
- administration of chemotherapy directly into the primary site organ (i.e. liver)

3. Preparation for insertion

Insertion is done by a physician in the operating room of a hospital. Placement is verified by x-ray prior to initiation of therapy.

4. Maintenance

- If the catheter tip is located in the epidural or intrathecal space the analgesic used (usually morphine) MUST be preservative free.
- When filling these pumps with medication, do not aspirate on the syringe. Medication remaining in the pump may be removed by holding the syringe down below the level of the body and allowing it to drain out via gravity.

- A special kit is used to access and fill the pump and the manufacturers directions should be followed in implementing the procedure.
- These pumps may remain in place indefinitely as long as they do not become infected.

L. *Epidural/Intrathecal Catheters*

1. Description

Epidural and Intrathecal catheters are open-ended catheters whose catheter distal tip is located in the intrathecal or epidural space.

2. Utilization

Epidural and Intrathecal catheters are generally utilized for the management of pain. Because the distal end of the catheter is located in the epidural or intrathecal space there are certain precautions that need to be followed:

- The analgesic used for these infusions (usually morphine) **MUST** be preservative free.
- Epidural and Intrathecal catheters are **NEVER** flushed with heparin solutions. If they need to be flushed use only sterile preservative free 0.9% NSS.
- Never aspirate on these catheters.
- If a PRN adapter is used on the end of the catheter, cleanse the adapter with a povidone-iodine swab or chlorhexidine prep (Chloraprep®) before injecting into the prn adapter (alcohol should never be used on these adapter or around the catheter because of the possible damage to the CNS if alcohol gets into the line).

3. Preparation for insertion

- Insertion of these catheters is done by a physician in the operating room of a hospital. This may be done on an out-patient basis. Placement is verified by x-ray prior to initiation of therapy.

4. Maintenance

- These catheters may remain in place indefinitely as long as they do not become infected.
- If a catheter is inadvertently pulled out, cover the exit site with a sterile gauze pad and notify the physician.
- The catheter may or may not be sutured in place depending on physician preference.

CHAPTER 12

Accessories

A. INFUSION PUMPS AND CONTROLLERS

There are too many makes and models of infusion pumps and controllers to attempt to describe their operation in detail. This section gives only a brief overview of various devices in common use, and their purposes. For detailed instructions on how to operate a device, read the manufacturer's booklet.

1. Advantages

Infusion pumps and controllers can regulate flow rates far more accurately than regulator clamps, and they don't have to be checked and reset as frequently. Controllers and certain types of pumps can deliver fluids much more slowly than manually regulated lines, and they may be used when small amounts of medication are to be administered over relatively long periods. Some pumps are useful for administering viscous fluids, such as blood and lipid emulsions (see Chapters 18 and 20). Finally, many devices contain safety features such as alarms when air gets in the line or a mechanical malfunction develops.

2. Disadvantages

Some models are fairly difficult to operate and monitor, and all require you to perform additional steps when starting an infusion.

Safety features may impart a false sense of security. Not all devices can be converted to gravity operation if they malfunction. Some older, heavier devices unnecessarily limit patients' mobility. Finally, the noise—especially in an intensive-care unit—may have an adverse psychological effect on patients.

3. Types Of Infusion Pumps And Controllers

a. **Syringe pumps (1-10psi)**—These devices can deliver small volumes of fluids very slowly (as little as 0.01 ml/hour) and are especially useful for purposes such as the following:

- Keeping a vein open
- Pediatric patients
- ICU/CCU settings
- Oxytocin infusion to induce labor (special models)
- Heparin administration during hemodialysis (special models)
- Cardiac catheterization (special models)
- Antibiotic infusions.
- Analgesic infusions

b. **Peristaltic pumps (5-15psi)**—There are two kinds of peristaltic pumps: linear and rotary. Certain older models require changing to a different size of tubing in order to adjust the flow rate, a process that increases the chances of contamination. Peristaltic pumps can deliver from 1 to 300ml/hour, and most models can be converted to gravity flow.

c. **Volumetric pumps (10-25psi)**—Volumetric pumps are the most accurate, with a delivery capacity ranging from 1 to 999 ml/hour. In general, volumetric pumps are more accurate than syringe and peristaltic pumps. However, because pumps exert a specific force, measured in pounds per square inch (PSI), the nurse must check the infusion site frequently for signs of infiltration. Most pumps will not alarm "occlusion" until a substantial amount of fluid has infiltrated the tissues. Another factor to consider in using a pump is the extra cost of the special cartridge and tubing required by most.

d. *Ambulatory pumps.* Ambulatory pumps vary in size and function and allow the patient a greater degree of mobility.

- Variable timed pumps may be programmed to deliver a specified amount of medication at designated intervals.
- TPN pumps may be programmed to deliver a specified amount of TPN solution and even allow the nurse to program in a designate tapering cycle for the TPN solution.
- Analgesic pumps allow the safe administration of an analgesic at a specified rate and generally allow for the programming of a specified bolus dose of the analgesic at designated intervals. (Patient controlled analgesic—PCA.)
- Continuous infusion ambulatory pumps are frequently used for hydration fluids or the administration of small amounts of medication over a prolonged period of time.
- Elastomeric pumps are designed for the administration of antibiotics, chemotherapy or other small (usually less than 400ml) of medications over a specified period of time. They look like a balloon inside a container. The flow rate is determined by the amount of fluid/ medication placed in the elastomeric device and the size of the device. The total amount of fluid/medication and the rate of flow is generally indicated on the top of the device. Elastomeric pumps are disposable, being used for only a single administration. They are easy to use, require no programming or special ancillary supplies and can be utilized by most patients with a minimal amount of teaching. To infuse the fluid/ medication at the designated rate the only requirement is to open the clamp that is attached to the tubing of the device. The device does not require an IV pole. It may be placed in the patients pocket, on the bed or a fanny pack (it does not require gravity to infuse).

e. *Infusion*—volume controllers. These devices work strictly by gravity. Their value lies in their greater simplicity and safety of operation relative to pumps and their much greater accuracy relative to manually operated clamps. Volume controllers generally deliver between 1 and 300 ml/hour. They cannot be used to deliver viscous fluids. The IV bottle or bag must be hung at least 1 meter above the insertion site, since a volume controller exerts no pumping action. However, since it works by gravity, a volume controller is generally safer to use than a pump. If an infiltration occurs, the flow through the volume controller will stop, more quickly than when a pump is used.

B. FILTERS

Filters come in different sizes and forms, but they all have one main purpose: to remove particles from IV fluids/medications. Particles may be in bits of solid material precipitated from the solution/container, bacteria, fungi, undissolved drug, or various other organic and inorganic impurities. You may want to consider using a filter when:

- Total parenteral nutrition is being given
- The patient is especially susceptible to infection (immunosuppressed)
- Filter is recommended for a specific drug

1. Types of filters

a. **Depth filters.** Depth filters remove particles of about 5 um or larger. Because of their construction, the pore size isn't uniform and no exact size rating is possible.

b. **Membrane filters** come in three pore sizes. The substance the filter is made of, as well as the pore size, determines what a filter can remove.

- 1 to 5 um—removes large particulate matter but does not remove bacteria
- 0.45 um—removes some bacteria and all particulate matter
- 0.22 um—removes all bacteria, fungi, yeast, and all particulate matter

c. **Needle/syringe filters**—These are membrane filters with a pore size of 0.45 to 5 um. They're used to filter medications before injection into an existing IV line or IV solution, especially when in-line filters are not used (see Chapter 13). After you draw up the medication into the syringe, discard the needle and filter (otherwise, you'll just inject the impurities into the IV line or solution). Attach a new sterile needle, prep the injection port on the tubing or solution with alcohol or povidone-iodine, and then inject the medication into the IV line or solution.

2. Air bubbles

Some membrane filters trap air, while others are air venting. When priming, it's especially important to flush out all air from the line, as any air that does get trapped in the filter will impede the flow of IV solution.

3. In-line vs. Add-on filters

Regardless of whether an in-line or add-on filter is used, follow the manufacturer's instructions for priming; some filters need to be inverted while priming, but some do not.

a. **IN-line filters**—In-line, or "final" filters are usually in the 0.22 to 0.45 um pore-size range. Because they're built into the tubing, a potential source of contamination is eliminated. The disadvantage of an in-line filter is that if an air bubble is trapped or if the filter becomes clogged with particulate matter, the entire tubing must be changed.

b. **Add-on filters**. The greatest disadvantage of an add-on filter is that it introduces two more potential points of contamination. The greatest advantage is flexibility.

4. Flow rate

A very-small-pore-size filter may slow the flow rate. You can partially counteract this effect by hanging the solution higher. Make sure you don't use a filter with a pore size so small that the proper rate of flow can't be maintained. Also, flow rates may begin to slow after the filter has hung for a period of time. This will be particularly noticeable if the patient is receiving multiple doses of medications through the line. The filter is performing its function and trapping all the particulate matter, thus clogging the filter and reducing the rate of flow. The filter and/or tubing must be changed if this should occur.

5. It is not necessary to add a filter on all IV fluids/ medications.

If you are using sterile fluids and connect the IV tubing, maintaining sterility of the line, there is no need to add a filter to the line. If your medications are mixed in the pharmacy, the compounding process is generally done under a laminar flow hood, and if you maintain the sterility of the system when attaching the tubing you do not need to add a filter to the line. If a medication requires a filter to be added the pharmacy will let you know and will generally supply you with the correct filter to use.

NOTE: Patients admitted to the emergency room, labor-and-delivery, those going to the operating room, or those experiencing life-threatening situations on the nursing units should not have IV lines started with a filter. These patients frequently need a "dump" of fluid, which may not be possible if there is a filter in-line.

CHAPTER 13

Additives And Admixtures

Patients who are being fed intravenously often receive their medications intravenously as well. IV additives can be given in a variety of ways: simultaneous infusion via a second set, intermittent infusion via a piggyback set or volume-control chamber, or admixture with the primary solution. In addition, medications can be injected directly (see Chapter 14).

A. SIMULTANEOUS INFUSION

1. Purpose

A second IV set is needed for continuous infusion of a solution simultaneously with a primary solution. The second set may be inserted into an injection port of the primary set, connected by means of a Y adapter or stopcock, for simultaneous infusion of two or more solutions. Never give incompatible substances simultaneously. If you are not sure whether two substances are compatible, check. If unable to ascertain their compatibility, do not infuse them simultaneously.

2. Equipment

To administer a medication or solution via a second set, you will need some or all of the following:

- ➤ Alcohol wipes
- ➤ Bottle/bag of second IV solution
- ➤ Second tubing

3. Procedure for simultaneous infusion

Figure 13-1 shows the setup for simultaneous infusion.

- ➤ Spike and hang the bottle/bag and prime the tubing (see chapter 6)
- ➤ Swap the injection port on the primary tubing with the alcohol wipe (scrub for 10-15 seconds). Use the lower port on the primary set, if there is more than one.
- ➤ Attach the distal end of the second IV tubing to the port on the primary set.
- ➤ Open the clamp on the second line, to make sure the solution is flowing feely, then adjust the flow to the ordered rate or attach the tubing to the infusion pump.
- ➤ Label the bottle/bag and tubing (see Chapter 15) and chart the procedure.

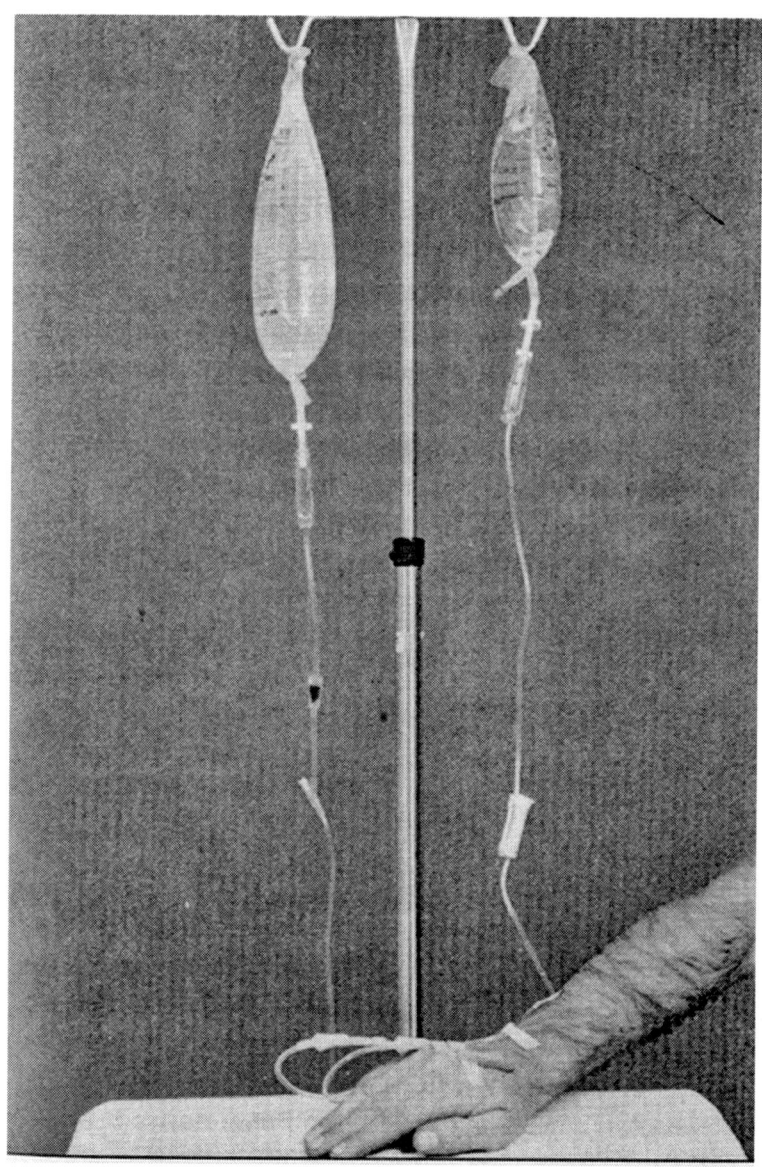

Figure 13-1. Simultaneous infusion

B. PIGGYBACK INFUSION

1. Purpose

A piggyback set is used for intermittent infusion of a medication. Intermittent infusion may be necessary to achieve peak blood levels of a medication, or to administer incompatible medications. If the second solution is incompatible with the primary one, flush the tubing with saline before attaching the piggyback to the primary line (see Chapter 15).

2. Equipment for gravity infusion

    a. ***Extension hook*** (usually comes packaged with the piggyback tubing)
    b. ***Bottle/bag of medication/solution***
    c. ***Alcohol wipes***
    d. ***Saline flush.*** If the two solutions are not compatible, you will also need a sterile 3-5ml syringe with sterile NSS

The procedure for flushing IV lines is outlined in Chapter 15.

3. Procedure for piggyback gravity infusion

    a. Hang the primary bottle/bag on an extension hook (usually provided in the bag/box with the secondary IV tubing. (Figure 13-2)
    b. Spike and hang the piggyback bottle/bag and prime the tubing (see Chapter 6).
    c. Swab the piggyback (upper, backcheck) port of the primary tubing with an alcohol wipe (10-15 seconds).
    d. If the two solutions are incompatible, flush the primary tubing below the injection port with saline (see Chapter 15).
    e. Attach the piggyback tubing to the primary IV tubing and regulate the flow of the piggyback fluid/medication to the ordered rate.
    e. Label the bottle/bag and tubing (see chapter 15) and chart the procedure.

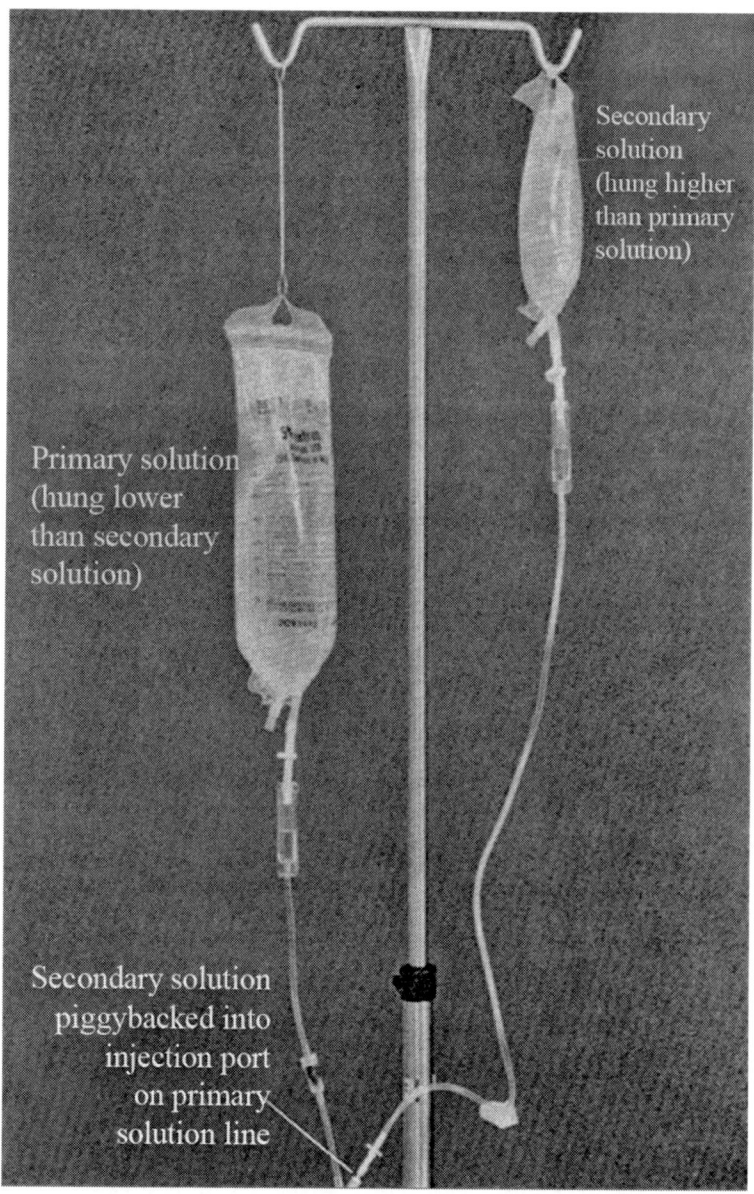

Figure 13-2

C. VOLUME-CONTROL CHAMBER

1. Purpose

A volume-control chamber, also called a fluid chamber, Burette, Volutrol, Soluset, or Buretrol, is used instead of a piggyback set for intermittent infusion when precise control of flow rate is necessary, as when a small amount of medication is to be infused over a long period. A volume-control set is often used as the primary line for infants and small children. (Figure 13-3)

2. Equipment—

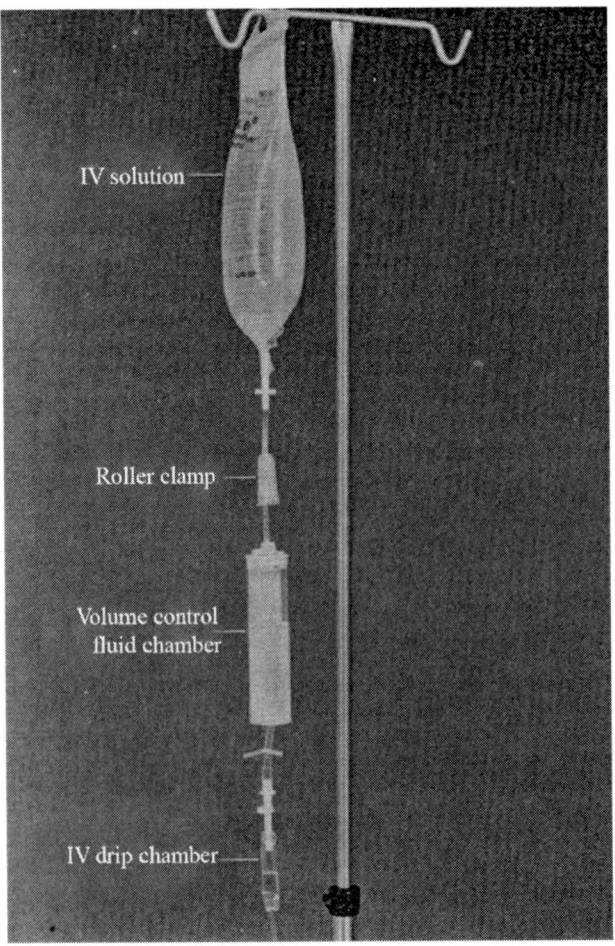

Figure 13-3

a. ***Additional equipment.*** The additional equipment is the same as for a simultaneous infusion (section A) except that the second tubing contains a volume-control chamber.

b. ***Drip rate.*** Most volume-control chambers are made to deliver 60 (microdrip) drops/ml.

c. ***Filters.*** Some volume-control chambers contain either a floating-valve filter or a membrane filter. The procedures for priming the drip chambers for the two types of filters are different. Consult the manufacturer's directions for priming these devices.

d. **Remaining procedure—if medication is to be added to the chamber/buretrol**

> ➢ Open the lower clamp, prime the tubing and close the clamp.
> ➢ Swab the injection port of the fluid chamber (Buretrol) with an alcohol wipe (10-15 seconds).
> ➢ Inject the prescribed medication into the volume control fluid chamber.
> ➢ Open the upper clamp, let the prescribed amount of solution run into the volume control fluid chamber and close the clamp.
> ➢ Gently mix the medication and the solution.
> ➢ Swab the injection port on the primary line with an alcohol wipe (10-15 seconds) and attach the tubing to the lowest port on the primary line.
> ➢ Clamp off the primary line or set it at KVO.
> ➢ Set the lower clamp on the volume-control set at the prescribed flow rate.
> ➢ Label all bottles/bags appropriately (see Chapter 15) and chart the procedure.

NOTE: A volume-control infusion line may also be used as the primary IV line.

D. ADMIXTURE WITH PRIMARY SOLTUION

1. Purpose

By mixing one or more drugs with the primary solution, you avoid several possibilities of contamination and considerably simplify administration and maintenance of the infusion. Admixture is possible only with compatible substances that are to be infused at the same rate.

2. Equipment

For each medication you add to the IV solution, if your institution's pharmacy does not perform this function, you will need the following:

- ➤ Filter needle/syringe
- ➤ Small-gauge (large-bore) 1½-inch needle
- ➤ Prescribed amount of drug in correct diluent

Other devices, such as double-headed pins and ampoule transfer siphons, are available for specialized applications.

3. Procedure

a. Injecting medication before spiking.

Again, the first four steps are increasingly performed by hospital pharmacies, which are better equipped than nursing stations.

- ➤ Draw the medication into the syringe
- ➤ Discard the needle and filter and replace with a small-gauge 1½-inch needle
- ➤ Remove the cap from the bottle/bag and swab the stopper with alcohol
- ➤ Inject the medication into the bottle/bag through the stopper and mix gently
- ➤ Before you administer the medication, inspect the solution for cloudiness, particles, color change, foaming, and other signs that something is wrong
- ➤ Label the bottle/bag (see Chapter 15) and chart the procedure

b. Injecting medication into a hanging bottle/bag.

Always make sure there is enough solution in the hanging container to dilute the drug sufficiently. If there is not, hang a fresh container. Always swab the injection port with alcohol before injecting the medication. And always clamp off the tubing before you inject any drug; otherwise the patient may receive a bolus of the drug.

➢ Nonvented bottle—remove the vent on the tubing, inject the medication into the vent port, and replace the vent (do not touch either end of the vent)

➢ Vented bottle—inject the medication into the triangle on the stopper

➢ Bag—inject the medication into the injection port and mix the solution gently by agitating the bottle/bag; do not pull on the tubing

➢ Label the bottle/bag (see Chapter 15) and chart the procedure

CHAPTER 14

Direct IV Injection

Certain drugs work best when injected directly into the vein rather than infused, whether or not the patient has an IV infusion running at the time. Medication may be injected rapidly or slowly, over a period of several minutes, through a variety of routes. The route depends partly on whether the medication is compatible with the primary solution. State and institutional regulation may prohibit IV injections by nurses who are not members of special teams or units (see Chapter 24), or may permit nurses to inject only certain drugs intravenously.

A. INJECTION DIRECTLY INTO A VEIN

IV medications may be injected directly into a vein, by IV bolus or push, when it is important for the patient to receive a large dose of medication fast, when the patient does not have an infusion running, or when it is impractical to inject medication through an existing line.

> ➤ IV bolus: The manual administration directly into a vein or IV tubing at a rate of 1 ml/30 seconds or less
> ➤ IV push: The manual administration directly into a vein or IV Tubing at a rate of 1ml/minute or greater.

1. Equipment

    a. *Rapid injection (IV bolus).* For injection all at once or very rapidly, you will need:

> Tourniquet
> Filter needle/syringe or prefilled syringe supplied by a drug manufacturer
> Straight needle or winged needle
> Povidone-iodine or alcohol wipe
> Sterile gauze pad

b. *Prolonged injection (IV push).* An alternative to inserting a needle directly attached to the syringe is the use of a winged-needle unit with the catheter attached to the syringe. The winged needle, being smaller and steadier than the syringe needle, is less likely to damage or perforate the vein over a period of several minutes. Also because the tension is on the catheter rather than on your hand, a winged-needle unit is more comfortable for both you and the patient. For this procedure you will need:

> Tourniquet
> Filter needle/syringe or prefilled syringe supplied by a drug manufacturer
> Winged-needle set
> Povidone-iodine or alcohol wipe
> Sterile gauze pads
> Tape

2. Procedure

a. *Rapid injection (IV bolus)*

> Draw up the medication into the filter needle/syringe 'if not already supplied in a filled syringe
> Discard the needle and filter and replace with the straight needle or winged needle
> Choose a vein, cleanse the insertion site with povidone-iodine or alcohol, and wipe with a gauze pad
> Perform venipuncture as described in Chapter 8
> If you are using a winged needle, place a piece of tape over the wings to stabilize the device and inject the medication with slow, even pressure—do not force the plunger

> Observe the patient closely for signs of adverse reaction
> Remove the tape, if any
> Place a sterile gauze pad over the site as you withdraw the needle
> Press the pad gently on the insertion site for one minute or until bleeding stops
> Cover the site with a sterile gauze pad or Band-Aid and chart the procedure

b. *Prolonged injection (IV push)*

> Draw up the medication into the filter needle/syringe if not already supplied in a filled syringe
> Disconnect and discard the needle and filter and attach the syringe to the catheter of the winged-needle set
> Choose a vein and prep the insertion site as described above
> Perform venipuncture as described in Chapter 8
> Flatten the wings of the needle and place a piece of tape over the wings to stabilize the device and inject the medication with a slow, even pressure—do not force the plunger

B. INJECTION THROUGH LOWER PORT OF TUBING

1. Purpose

This is the most common route, and the easiest to use, in patients who already have an IV infusion. (Figure 14-1) Incompatible medications can be given directly into the IV line as long as the tubing is flushed with saline before and after the injection of the incompatible substance (see Chapter **15**).

2. Equipment

> Filter needle/syringe
> Prescribed medication
> 2 syringes with 3-5ml of NSS each
> Alcohol wipes

3. Procedure

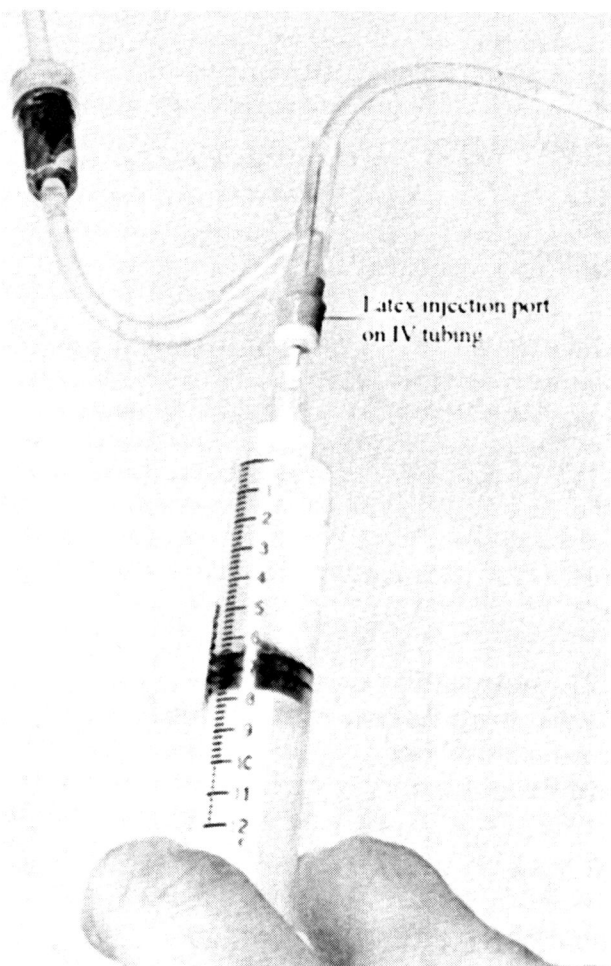

Figure 14-1. Push into injection port on IV tubing

> Draw up the appropriate amount of medication with a filter needle/syringe
> Discard the filter needle
> Swab (10-15 seconds) the lower injection port on the primary IV tubing
> Clamp off the tubing above the injection port on the primary IV
> If necessary, flush the tubing with 3-5ml NSS (see Chapter 15)

➢ Attach the syringe with the medication, aspirate for blood then slowly inject the IV medication.
➢ Flush the primary line again with 3-5ml of NSS
➢ Open the clamp and regulate the flow rate
➢ Chart the procedure

C. INJECTION THROUGH A HEPARIN/SALINE LOCK OR INTERMITTENT INFUSION ADAPTER

1. Purpose

A heparin/saline lock is used when a patient needs intermittent infusion or slow injection of medication but does not require a constant infusion. It keeps the vein open by preventing clotting but has the added advantage of allowing the patient greater mobility than a continuous hookup and of reducing the risk of fluid overload. A heparin/saline lock can also be used for drawing blood samples. (Figure 14-2)

Note: Explain to the patient why he/she will have the device inserted, and make sure the patient understands that it must be kept clean and dry and intact.

2. Equipment

A standard winged-needle set or CON can be converted to a heparin/saline lock by inserting a special prn adapter. If you have a choice, a CON is preferable to a winged-needle device.

➢ Tourniquet
➢ Winged-needle or CON device
➢ Intermittent infusion adapter (prn adapter)
➢ Sterile dressing (transparent dressings are preferred)
➢ Alcohol wipes or chlorohexidine prep
➢ Tape
➢ Syringe with 3-5ml of NSS or 3-5ml 1:10 or 1:100 units/ml heparin flush solution (flushing solutions of saline vs. heparin are generally determined by your facility).

3. Starting a heparin/saline lock

a. Choose a vein and prep the patient as described in Chapter 7

b. If an extension tubing is attached to the prn adapter, wipe the prn adapter injection port with an alcohol wipe and flush the line with NSS

c. With the winged-needle or CON device, perform the venipuncture as described in Chapter 8 and check for a blood return

d. Withdraw the needle (stylet) from the CON device or detach the venting plug from the winged-needle device, and attach the prn adapter to the hub of the CON or winged needle

e. Tape the device securely

f. Wipe the prn adapter injection port with an alcohol wipe and inject 3-5ml of NSS or heparin flush solution

g. If a medication is to be injected, flush with NSS then slowly inject the ordered medication followed by another flush with NSS after the medication has been administered (if it is your facility policy the heparin flush solution is administered after the NSS flush following the medication administration)

h. Label the site and chart the procedure

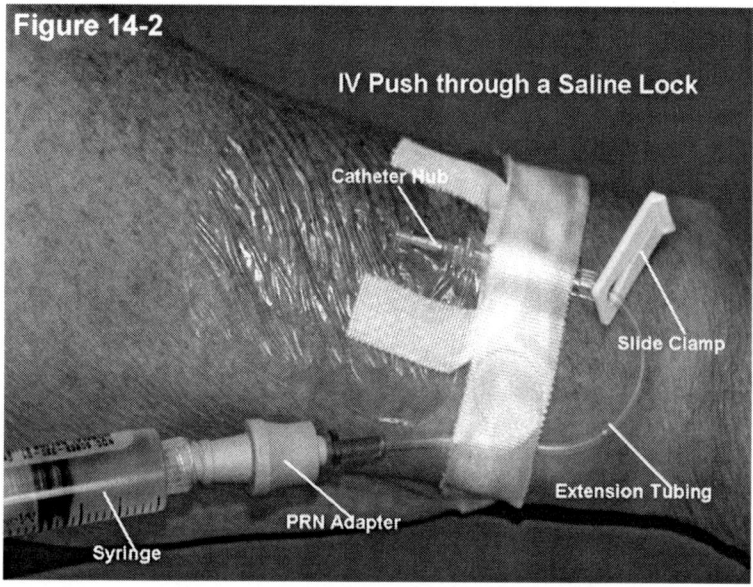

Figure 14-2

IV Push through a Saline Lock

Catheter Hub

Slide Clamp

Extension Tubing

PRN Adapter

Syringe

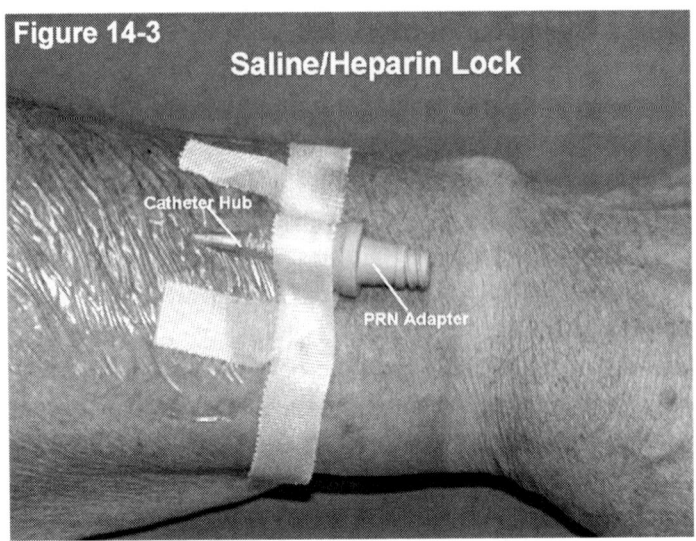

4. Administering medications by means of a heparin/saline lock

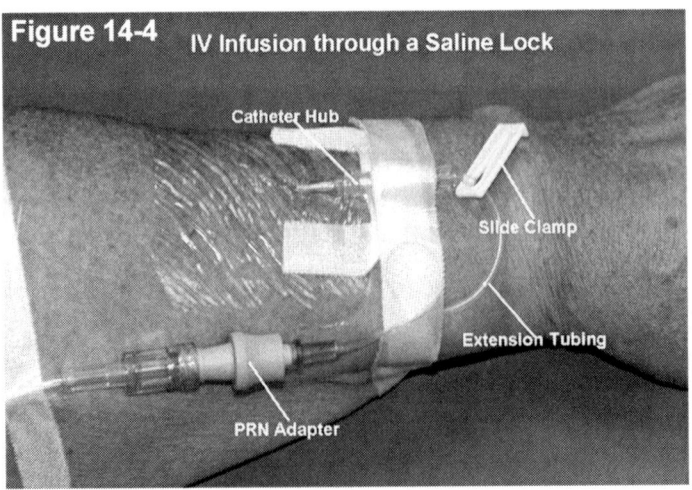

a. Injection

Swab the prn adapter injection port with alcohol (10-15 seconds)

> Draw up the medication in a syringe

- ➢ Obtain a 3-5ml syringe with NSS for flushing
- ➢ Obtain a 3-5ml syringe with a heparin flush solution (1:10 or 1:100 units of heparin) According to your facility's policy
- ➢ Insert the NSS syringe into the injection port on the prn adapter and aspirate for blood
- ➢ Flush the adapter with the NSS and remove the syringe from the adapter
- ➢ Swab the injection port with an alcohol wipe
- ➢ Insert the syringe with the medication into the injection port on the prn adapter and inject the medication at the prescribed rate
- ➢ Remove the medication syringe from the adapter
- ➢ Swab the injection port on the prn adapter with an alcohol wipe
- ➢ Attach the NSS flush syringe to the prn adapter and flush (repeat the injection of NSS for each drug to be administered)
- ➢ Observe the patient for possible signs and symptoms of drug reaction
- ➢ Chart the procedure

b. *Infusion.*

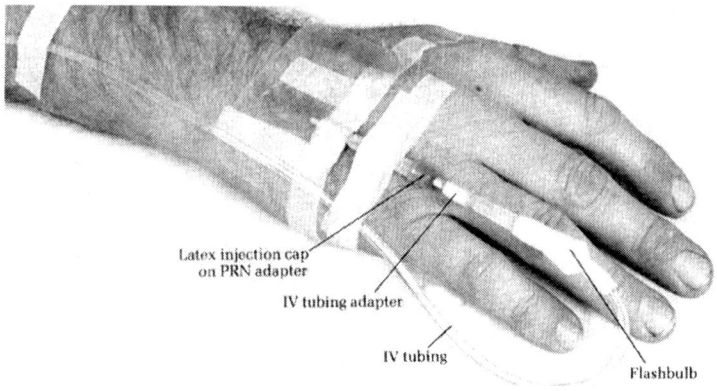

Latex injection cap on PRN adapter

IV tubing adapter

IV tubing

Flashbulb

Figure 14-5

- ➢ Set up the necessary equipment and prime it as described in Chapter 6

> Swab the injection port on the prn adapter with alcohol (10-15 seconds)
> Draw up 3-5ml of NSS in a syringe
> Insert the syringe into the injection port on the adapter and aspirate for blood
> Flush the adapter with the saline and remove the syringe
> Swab the injection port with alcohol
> Attach the IV tubing to the prn adapter injection port
> Regulate the flow rate
> Label the bottle/bag appropriately and chart the procedure
> After the infusion has ended, detach the IV administration set, flush the adapter with 3-5ml of NSS, followed by a heparin flush if indicated by your facility's policy

D. ADVANTAGES OF DIRECT IV INJECTION

The advantages of direct IV injection are:

> Immediate peak blood levels may be achieved
> It is fast and easy to administer, particularly in an emergency situation
> Less fluid volume is required than for IV piggyback or primary solution
> It may be given if PO or IM route is contraindicated
> It may be the desired route if the drug would be incompatible with other IV drugs or solution being infused

E. DISADVANTAGES OF DIRECT IV INJECTION

The disadvantages of direct IV injection include the following:

> Immediate peak blood levels may be achieved—the entire dose is on board and, consequently, reactions will tend to be more severe

> It may cause venous irritation—many of the drugs are fairly concentrated and irritate the vein intima
> It may be time consuming—IV push drugs may take several minutes to administer
> If a patient's circulatory system is compromised (i.e., in an arrest), the risk of intra-arterial injection is greatly increased ("normal" landmarks and distinguishing signs are absent); observation must be intensified to prevent serious consequences
> The medication cannot be given by direct IV injection if it needs to be diluted in a large amount of solute. It would then be best to give the drug by primary or piggyback infusion.

F. POSSIBLE COMPLICATIONS OF DIRECT IV INJECTION

1. Drugs that frequently cause severe reaction

   a. CNS depressants. These include tranquilizers, analgesics, narcotics
   b. Anti-inflammatory agents
   c. Anesthetics
   d. Antibiotics
   e. Antineoplastics
   f. Anticonvulsants

2. Possible side effects

   a. *Cardiac arrhythmias*
   b. *GI upset.* With some drugs, this may be an early warning of reaching toxic levels.
   c. *CNS depression.* Side effects include drowsiness, mental confusion, hypotension, respiratory depression.
   d. *GU symptoms*
   e. *Neurological symptoms*
   f. *Extravasation.* Some of the drugs that are particularly irritating to soft tissues on infiltration include:

   > Dopamine
   > Dilantin

> Mannitol
> Valium
> Phenobarbital
> Digoxin
> Dextrose (greater than 10%)
> Anti-inflammatory agents
> Antineoplastics
> Vasoconstrictors

G. ANTIDOTES

Antidotes for various drug reactions due to direct injection include:

> Diphenhydramirie (Benadryl)—for allergic rash or phenothiazine reaction
> Epinephrine—for allergic anaphylactoid respiratory reactions
> Phentolamine (Regitine)—for adverse reaction to vasoconstrictors
> Naloxone (Narcan)—for reaction to narcotics
> Protamine sulfate—for reaction to heparin
> Antineoplastics reaction—sodium thiosulfate for mechlorethamine (Mustargen); sodium bicarbonate for doxorubicin (Adriamycin); hyaluronidase (Wydase) for vincristine (Oncovin) and vinblastine (Velban).

H. BASIC CONSIDERATIONS

The basic considerations for administering any drug directly into a patient's venous system must include:

1. Application of the five R's

> Right patient
> Right drug
> Right dose
> Right route
> Right time

2. Knowledge of the patient's condition and medical history

> ➤ Be aware of the patient's condition before administering the medication.
> ➤ Know the patient's history, allergies, and/or possible contraindications before using the drug (e.g., propranolol (Inderal) is indicated for the treatment of tachycardia but is contraindicated for use with asthmatic patients).

3. Following correct procedure

Follow correct procedure (as stated earlier in this chapter), utilizing aseptic technique.

CHAPTER 15

Compatibility Of IV Solutions

This chapter cannot begin to list all drug and IV solution incompatibilities; that would take a book in itself. Rather, here are some general guidelines to follow. For information about specific drugs and IV solutions, you may consult reference sources such as those listed in section D.

A. LABELING

Whenever you add medication to an IV solution, you must label the bottle/bag with the following pertinent information:

> ➤ Name of patient
> ➤ Patient's ID or hospital number Patient's room number and bed
> ➤ Name of medication
> ➤ Amount and strength of medication
> ➤ Expiration date of medication
> ➤ Diluent or reconstitution medium, if any
> ➤ Date and time medication was added
> ➤ Name of IV solution Flow rate
> ➤ Your name or initials as required by institutional policy

B. TYPES OF INCOMPATIBILITIES

There are a limited number of references on intravenous incompatibilities (see section D), and much remains unknown. For those reasons, it is critical for the nurse to understand some of the basic or underlying mechanisms of incompatibilities and to be able to identify potential problems that can be researched for more definitive answers or referred to the IV admixture pharmacy service, if one exist, in the institution. Intravenous incompatibilities may result from undesirable chemical or physical phenomena when two or more intravenous medications come into contact with each other. In general, incompatibilities can be divided into two categories, therapeutic and pharmaceutical. Pharmaceutical incompatibilities can be further divided into physical and chemical categories.

1. Therapeutic incompatibilities

Therapeutic incompatibilities result when two or more incompatible drugs are combined, which produces a response completely different in nature or in intensity from that expected. An example of such a reaction is in the mixture of an aminoglycoside (gentamicin) and a penicillin (carbenicillin, ticarcillin) in the same bottle or in the infusion of the two drugs simultaneously in the same primary tubing. A chemical reaction between the two drugs results, causing inactivation of the aminoglycoside and thus preventing the patient from receiving the full benefit of the antibiotic. A more general example deals with the combination of a bacteriostatic and a bactericidal antibiotic. Whether these antibiotics are infused together or separately, a therapeutic incompatibility results, not from the chemical characteristics of each drug, but from their pharmacologic effects. A bacteriostatic antibiotic (e.g., chloramphenicol) inhibits bacterial growth whereas a bactericidal antibiotic (e.g., penicillin) kills bacteria. Since bactericidal antibiotics are only effective against multiplying bacteria, bacteriostatic antibiotics may inhibit the antibacterial effect of the bactericidal antibiotic.

2. Pharmaceutical incompatibilities

a. *Physical incompatibilities.* Physical incompatibilities may result from the inability of a drug to dissolve in a solution or from the combination of two drugs, which forms a complex or precipitate that is insoluble and is visualized as a precipitate or haze. On occasion such a reaction may result in a color change of the solution or evolution of gas in the admixture. Examples of physical incompatibilities are Valium mixed in D5W and phenytoin sodium added to an aqueous solution with an acidic pH.

b. *Chemical incompatibilities.* Chemical incompatibilities result from reactions that are often manifested in both a physical and a therapeutic incompatibility. A chemical incompatibility may result in a therapeutic incompatibility without the formation of visual physical evidence. An example is the hydrolysis of drugs (Penicillin in water is eventually inactivated without visual evidence). The chemical reaction between acidic and basic drugs is the most common source of chemical incompatibility. Such a combination may result in a new pH of the solution and a consequent instability of one of the drugs. Examples include ampicillin in D5W stored at room temperature for more than four hours prior to administration and the oxidation of epinephrine in alkaline solutions when exposed to light.

C. GENERAL GUIDELINES

1. Diluent

Does the medication have its own diluent, as do drugs such as diazepam (Valium)? If it does, it is probably incompatible with other medications or IV solutions.

2. Printed precautions

Does the package insert or label contain precautions on mixing the medication, as with drugs such as erythromycin lactobionate (Erythrocin Lactobionate-IV) or nitroprusside (Nipride)? If so, read the directions carefully.

3. Colloids

Colloids like amphotericin B (Fungizone) are likely to "salt out" (precipitate) in the presence of electrolytes such as sodium chloride (saline) and bacteriostatic agents such as benzyl alcohol.

4. Blood

Never mix blood or blood products with anything. The protein in blood may bind to other agents and destroy their effectiveness. Even more important, you risk coagulation or lysis of the cells.

5. Antibiotics

   a. ***Drug interactions.*** Try to avoid mixing antibiotics in the same solution, as they are likely to interact. For example, tetracyclines interfere with the bactericidal action of penicillins; carbenicillin or ticarcillin inactivates gentamicin or tobramycin.

   b. ***Hydrolysis.*** Does the medication look, smell, or sound like one of the penicillins—for example, ampicillin (Alpen-N, Amcill-S, Penbritin-S, Polycillin-N), carbenicillin (Geopen, Pyopen), or methicillin (Dimocillin, Staphcillin)? These antibiotics are easily hydrolyzed by either acids or bases.

6. Calcium

Calcium is an electrolyte and is present in many commonly used parenteral solutions (e.g., lactated Ringer's solution). At an alkaline pH it will be precipitated out of Solution, especially when drugs such as cephalothin sodium (Keflin), sodium bicarbonate, and potassium phosphate are added to the solution.

7. Mixing intravenous admixtures (acidity and alkalinity)

Add one drug at a time to the large-volume parenteral solution, mix it thoroughly, and then examine it visually. Some visual incompatibilities are concentration dependent and may require a certain amount of time or concentration before appearing. It is a good idea to add the most concentrated or most soluble additive to the solution first. The more dilute the drug is, the less likely that acid-base interactions will occur. Any medication with a very high pH (alkaline) or low pH (acid) is likely to cause compatibility problems.

8. Precipitates

Some precipitates are very fine and dispersed, making them very difficult to detect. This is especially true if the solution is colored, as when multivitamins or riboflavin are added. In such cases, add the color-producing drug last in order to be able to visualize the solution. For example, Valium added to a large-volume parenteral is very critical. If Valium's solubility is exceeded, the fine yellow color of multivitamins may mask the Valium precipitate if Valium is added to the solution first.

9. Phenol Red

An orange solution that is not a vitamin may contain phenol red, which is sensitive to alkaline pH. It may not be disconcerting to you to mix an additive containing phenol red (e.g., potassium chloride, magnesium chloride, or calcium chloride) with a compatible basic drug (e.g., ampicillin), but the resulting magenta color may create panic among patients, physicians, and other nurses.

10. Rules of thumb

a. Pharmacologic groups of drugs (families) usually react in a similar manner. If you know of an incompatibility with one drug, most likely the same is true for the other drugs in that group.

b. If you are not sure about the compatibility of drugs to be mixed, do not proceed before either contacting someone who can provide you with an answer or researching an answer yourself. If you are unable to find out about the compatibility, do not mix them.

D. SOURCES OF INFORMATION ON DRUG COMPATIBILITY

Your pharmacist should be a good source of information. Alternatively, you may consult published materials such as the following:

> ➢ American Hospital Formulary Service
> ➢ *Drug Interactions Index* by William Norcross and Robert T. Weibert (PMIC, 1988)
> ➢ *Physicians' Desk Reference* (Medical Economics; published yearly)

E. FLUSHING IV LINES

1. Purpose

Flushing helps prevent incompatible substances from coming into contact with each other. Flush with sterile nonpyrogenic normal saline 0.9% (NSS) after each incompatible medication you inject through the IV tubing or the intermittent-infusion prn adapter. Flushing also helps to maintain the patency of a heparin or saline lock.

2. Equipment

> ➢ Sterile syringe containing 3-5ml of NSS (or 3-5ml of a heparin flush solution 1:10 or 1:100 units/ml)
> ➢ Alcohol wipes

3. Procedure

> ➢ Swab the injection port on the prn adapter with alcohol (10-15 seconds)
> ➢ Attach the syringe with the saline or heparin flush solution to the prn adapter
> ➢ Aspirate for blood

➤ Inject the saline, or heparin flush, solution through the prn adapter (do not force it)
➤ If necessary you may aspirate and flush again
➤ Detach the syringe from the prn adapter
➤ If unable to aspirate blood from the IV line you may need to use Alteplase (see Chapter 11) to open the line

CHAPTER 16

Changing And Discontinuing IV Infusions

When handling IV equipment, maintain sterile technique at all times. If you have any doubt about the sterility of any piece of equipment, discard it.

A. *CHANGING IV SOLUTION CONTAINERS*

1. Frequency

Change containers at least every 24 hours, and more often according to a physician's orders. It is not necessary to wait for the bottle/bag to be emptied of the last drop of solution before you change it.

2. Procedure

For spiking and priming technique, see Chapter 6.

> ➢ Make sure the drip chamber under the old container is at least half full
> ➢ Close the regulator clamp to a KVO rate
> ➢ Remove the protective cap from the new container. If using a bottle, wipe the rubber stopper on the bottle with an alcohol wipe
> ➢ Remove the old container from the IV pole

➢ Remove the spike from the old container and insert it in the new one
➢ Hang the new container and label it
➢ Regulate the flow rate
➢ Drain any remaining solution from the old container and discard it in the proper receptacle
➢ Chart the procedure

B. CHANGING IV ADMINISTRATION SETS AND DRESSINGS

1. Frequency

Change tubing on a continuous IV every 72 hours, change tubing on intermittent IV's, TPN, PPN and Dextrose greater than 5% every 24 hrs. Change tubing on blood after 2 units. If possible, time the tubing change to coincide with changes of containers, needles or catheter. However, if a patient is admitted with an IV already running, you may need to connect new tubing and a new container to the catheter/needle already in place. Change gauze dressings every 24-48 hours, or sooner, if they become wet or contaminated. If transparent dressings are used, they need to be changed every 72 hours and prn for a peripheral line and once a week for central lines, and prn (if the dressing becomes wet or contaminated).

2. Procedure

➢ Close the regulator clamp on the new tubing
➢ Remove the protective cover or cap from the new container. If a bottle is used, wipe the stopper with an alcohol wipe
➢ Spike the container
➢ Hang the new container and prime the tubing (see Chapter 6)
➢ If the dressing is to be changed, hold the catheter needle in place with one hand and remove the old dressing from the IV site, being careful not to dislodge or wiggle the catheter/needle unnecessarily
➢ Cleanse the insertion site with Chlorohexidine Gluconate solution (Chloraprep®) or an alcohol wipe followed by

a povidone-iodine wipe may be used (according to your facility's policy). Let the solution air dry on the patient's skin.

➢ Place a large sterile gauze pad or alcohol wipe under the hub and adapter
➢ Close the regulator clamp on the old IV tubing
➢ With one hand holding the catheter/needle, grasp the hub and carefully remove the old tubing adapter
➢ Remove the protective cap from the new tubing and attach the new adapter to the hub
➢ Remove the gauze pad or alcohol wipe and clean the area of any blood or fluid that may have spilled during the procedure
➢ Apply a new dressing
➢ Loop the tubing and tape it to the patient's skin. Regulate the flow rate
➢ Label the new container, tubing, and dressing
➢ Drain any remaining solution from the old container and tubing and discard them in the designated receptacle along with the old dressing
➢ Chart the procedure

C. CHANGING IV CATHETERS AND NEEDLES

Unless the patient is running short of acceptable new sites, a peripheral IV infusion should be moved every 48-72 hours. This, of course, involves a completely new prep, venipuncture, and infusion start, which are covered in Chapters 7, 8, and 9 respectively. If the site needs to be extended beyond the 72 hours because of limited venous access, the physician should be notified and an order for the infusion to continue at that site should be obtained and documented in the patient's record. The infusion site should then be watched even more closely. the condition of the site documented and the IV removed at the first sign of irritation, infiltration, and/or phlebitis.

D. CHANGING STOPCOCKS

Stopcocks should be changed every 24 to 72 hours, at the same time the tubing is changed. If you change the tubing because you suspect it is contaminated, you must also change the stopcock. Once the injection-port cover is removed from the stopcock, consider the port contaminated; do not use it again.

E. DISCONTINUING AN INFUSION

1. Routine removal

➢ Remove the outer tape and the dressing
➢ Stabilize the catheter/needle with one hand and carefully remove the tape (avoid moving the catheter/needle inside the vein)
➢ Press gently on the puncture site with a sterile gauze pad
➢ Slowly withdraw the catheter/needle in line with the vein (see Figure 16-1)

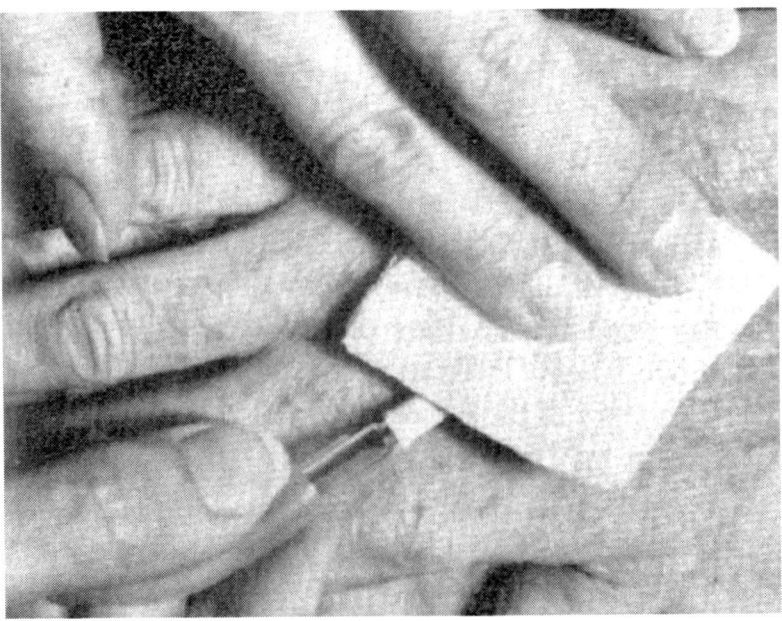

Figure 16-1. Discontinuing an infusion

➢ Press firmly on the site with the gauze pad for at least 30 seconds, or until bleeding stops, to avoid a hematoma. You may elevate the limb during the time digital pressure is being applied

➤ Cover the site with a sterile gauze pad or bandage and chart the procedure

➤ Empty any remaining solution from the container and tubing and discard them, along with the dressing and catheter/needle, in the designated receptacles

2. Removal when there is a problem with the infusion

a. ***Failure to flow well.*** Try to reestablish good flow by techniques like this:

➤ Repositioning the catheter
➤ Squeezing the tubing
➤ Hanging the bottle/bag higher
➤ Flushing with saline and aspirating

If a filter is used, it may be clogged and thus need to be changed. If necessary, get help from someone more experienced—such as your institution's IV team.

b. ***Infiltration or clotting.*** If you are unable to reestablish good flow by any of the methods recommended above, suspect infiltration or a clot in the catheter—even if no signs of these problems are evident. If you suspect the site may have been infiltrated with a drug that could be damaging to the soft tissues, close the regulator clamp on the IV tubing but do not remove the catheter! needle. Contact the IV therapy specialist on duty or the pharmacist for possible action. If the infiltration involves a plain solution or medication that will not damage soft tissues, discontinue the infusion at once and start again in another vein.

c. ***Redness, soreness, or phlebitis.*** If an IV site is red, sore, or phlebitic, the line must be discontinued. If a bacterial infection is suspected, culture the site (see Chapter 21) before discontinuing the infusion. If necessary, call on someone more experienced for help. To assist in the healing process and make the patient more comfortable, apply warm, moist compresses to the area.

d. **Charting and follow-up.** Chart any problems you find when discontinuing an infusion, and alert the appropriate personnel as to the need for continued observation of the puncture site.

F. DISPOSAL OF USED EQUIPMENT

All used IV equipment, from the bottle/bag on down, is contaminated. Therefore, you cannot just drop it in the nearest wastebasket. For the protection of curious visitors and of all personnel who participate in waste disposal, used IV equipment must be discarded in special receptacles.

1. Bottles, bags, and tubing

These should be drained and placed in the designated receptacle.

2. Needles

- ➤ Needles should NOT be broken, bent, or otherwise manipulated
- ➤ Place all needles in a puncture proof container designed for that purpose
- ➤ If you accidentally stick yourself with a contaminated needle, notify your supervisor immediately

3. Syringes

- ➤ Syringes should be placed in puncture proof containers along with the needles
- ➤ Needles and syringes should be disposed of according to your state's hazardous waste disposal regulations (incineration is the preferred method of disposal)

CHAPTER 17

Monitoring IV Infusions

Many things can go wrong with an IV infusion. Some complications of IV therapy can quickly become fatal. That is why it is important to check infusions frequently—at least every two hours, and more often if a hypertonic solution or a drug is being infused or if the patient is very young, old, or debilitated.

A. PROBLEMS WITH FLOW RATE

1. Runaway IV

    a. *What may happen.* A clamp may slip, or the patient or a visitor may open a clamp. The resulting too-rapid infusion might not do harm, but it could have drastic, even fatal, consequences:

> ➤ Circulatory overload, leading to congestive heart failure and pulmonary edema
> ➤ Toxic overdose of a medication infused faster than the body can metabolize it

    b. *Intervention.* If you observe signs of congestive heart failure or pulmonary edema—rapid, labored breathing, rapid pulse, increased blood pressure, distended neck veins—slow the infusion to its minimum rate, place the patient in high Fowler's position, and call a physician. If you observe signs of shock or anaphylaxis, replace the infusion with normal (0.9%) saline at a KVO rate, and call a physician. The saline infusion keeps the vein open and helps counteract the effects of shock on the circulatory volume.

c. *Suggestions for prevention*

> Know your patient's cardiovascular status and medical history.
> Monitor your patient's intake and output carefully. Notify the physician if your patient appears unable to handle the fluid volume.
> Check the IV infusion often for correct flow rate.

2. Obstructed or irregular flow

a. *What may happen.* A solution may refuse to flow at the prescribed rate, or may stop entirely, for any of several reasons:

> The tourniquet may have been left on the patient's arm
> The catheter/needle may be pushed against the vein wall
> The tubing may be kinked or pinched in a side rail
> The bottle/bag may not be hanging high enough
> The tubing may be clamped too tightly
> The patient may have shifted position or be lying on the tubing
> The tape over the tubing may be too tight
> If a volume-control chamber is being used, air may be trapped in the filter, the filter may be wet, or both vents may be closed
> If an infusion pump or volume controller is being used, it may have been set up incorrectly or may be malfunctioning
> There may be clotting or infiltration at the insertion site (for details, see section B)
> The air vent may be occluded (wet)
> The roller slide clamp may be closed

*b. **Intervention.*** Examine the entire setup, beginning with the tourniquet (which should be promptly removed) and then proceeding from the bottle/bag down to the puncture site. If you cannot find the problem, ask someone more experienced—such as your institution's IV team—for help.

*c. **Suggestions for prevention***

> ➤ Do not place any constricting device (e.g., restraints) over or directly above an IV site.
> ➤ Check the infusion system regularly.

3. Improper flow rate

*a. **What may happen.*** The regulator clamp may have slipped or been tampered with, or it may have been set incorrectly initially.

*b. **Intervention.*** Resist the temptation to "catch up" by setting the flow rate faster than the rate prescribed. Also resist the temptation to set the flow rate fast in order to use up the contents of the container. It is better to start a new container and to make sure the clamp is set to permit the correct flow rate.

*c. **Suggestions for prevention***

> ➤ Calculate the flow rate accurately
> ➤ Check the system regularly for the prescribed rate of flow

B. PROBLEMS AT THE INSERTION SITE

1. Extravasation (infiltration)

*a. **What may happen.*** The catheter/needle may have been pulled partly or entirely out of the vein, flooding the surrounding tissue with IV solution. The catheter! needle may have perforated the opposite wall of the vein, or the patient's movements may have widened the opening in the vein, causing the contents—blood and IV solution—to leak into the surrounding tissues. Signs of infiltration include these:

- ➢ Swelling
- ➢ Pain
- ➢ Coolness
- ➢ Slight, or no, blood return

The consequences of infiltration range from mild and temporary to severe and lasting, and include pain, loss of use of other veins in the infiltrated limb, and permanent damage to nerves. Extravasation of irritation solutions and/or medications may cause necrosis of tissues, and disfigurement or loss of the limb.

b. Intervention

- ➢ Discontinue the infusion.
- ➢ Using a new venipuncture device, start the infusion at another site.
- ➢ If an irritating solution and/or medication is involved, contact the IV therapy specialist, the physician, or the pharmacist for possible treatment before discontinuing the line.
- ➢ Apply warm, moist compresses for a 20-minute period three or four times a day to ease discomfort at the old site.
- ➢ Apply cool compresses if the infiltrated solution and/or medication will irritate or damage soft tissue.

c. Suggestions for prevention

- ➢ Use a hand board or arm board to stabilize the catheter/needle when the site is over a joint or the patient is especially active.
- ➢ Palpate the site frequently to check for signs of coolness or swelling of the tissues.
- ➢ Check the site regularly—and especially before infusing medications—for good blood return.

2. Local infection

a. What may happen. Bacteria may enter the puncture wound by migrating along the skin tract, or contamination may

occur due to poor aseptic technique on insertion or poor site maintenance. The site will be sore, with varying degrees of warmth and redness. Foul-smelling, or purulent, drainage may be noted at the site.

b. Intervention

➢ Discontinue the infusion.

➢ Culture the catheter, site, and drainage according to your institution's policies and procedures.

➢ Clean the site with an antiseptic solution and cover it with a sterile dressing.

➢ Restart the IV infusion if necessary—preferably in the opposite limb.

➢ Notify the patient's physician.

➢ Chart the procedure and your observations in the patient's record.

c. Suggestions for prevention

➢ Maintain aseptic technique when starling an IV infusion.

➢ Keep all IV sites clean and dry.

➢ Be careful to avoid touch contamination when changing IV tubings, dressings, etc.

3. Clotting

a. What may happen? A fibrin sheath or fibrin flap may have formed around the catheter causing the IV to run slowly and you will be unable to withdraw blood from the line. Also, a thrombus may have formed within the catheter because of inadequate flow rate or flushing.

b. Intervention. You may try flushing the line with NSS (see Chapter 15) through the injection port on the tubing. Do not force the saline into the tubing, as you may dislodge the clot and push it into the circulatory system. If unable to re-establish patency of the peripheral line, discontinue the line and start the IV in a new location, preferably in the opposite limb. If unable to re-establish patency of a Central Venous Access Device, utilize the Alteplase (see Chapter 11) to clear the line.

c. *Suggestions for prevention*

> ➤ Check the IV frequently to make sure the tubing is not kinked.
> ➤ Be careful not to allow the IV to run "dry".
> ➤ Check the flow rate regularly.

4. Phlebitis

a. *What may happen.* Many things may actually cause phlebitis (the inflammation of a vein). They may be grouped into one of three categories:

> ➤ Mechanical phlebitis—the catheter/needle movement within the vein may actually irritate and inflame the intima of the vein, causing "mechanical" phlebitis.
> ➤ Chemical phlebitis—various drugs, especially cephalothin (Keflin), gentamicin (Garamycin), minocycline (Minocin), tetracycline (Achromycin), cefamandole (Mandol), potassium chloride, penicillin, and anesthetic agents, have been known to irritate and inflame the vein intima, causing "chemical" phlebitis.
> ➤ Bacterial phlebitis—microorganisms may contaminate the system anywhere along the line. Touch contamination while changing the IV solution or tubing, attaching a piggyback medication, manipulating a stopcock or CVP manometer, injecting into the line, or migration of bacteria along the skin tract into the puncture site may allow for the entrance of bacteria into the body, causing "bacterial" phlebitis. The severity of phlebitis may be categorized by degrees.

Watch for the corresponding signs:

> ➤ 1°—pain, soreness, or tenderness at the site, without redness.
> ➤ 2°—pain and soreness with redness at, or extending less than 3 inches above, the site.

> 3°—pain, soreness, and redness extending more than 3 inches above the site, and/or the presence of a palpable cord in the vein.
> 4°—pain, soreness, and redness extending more than three inches in length above the site, a palpable cord and/or evidence of exudate at the site.

b. Intervention. If the patient complains of pain while a medication is being infused, try continuing the infusion while applying warm, moist compresses to the limb. If, however, pain continues or increases and/or redness develops, discontinue the infusion and start again elsewhere, if possible in the opposite limb. If you suspect a drug is causing the inflammation, can you administer it in a larger quantity of solution so that it is more dilute? Or can you administer it over a shorter period of time? Carefully watch the old site for signs of infection; culture it according to your institution's policies, particularly if you suspect bacterial phlebitis. Apply warm, moist compresses to the area to help with the healing process. Chart your observations in the patient's record.

c. Suggestions for prevention

> Check the site frequently for signs of soreness or redness.
> Infuse the medication at the prescribed rate of flow.
> Use the smallest-size catheter/needle that will meet the patient's needs and allow for adequate dilution of the solution and/or medication in the vein.
> Dilute irritating medications with as much diluent as possible.

5. Thrombophlebitis

a. What may happen. Thrombophlebitis is a complication of phlebitis. When the wall of the vein becomes irritated and inflamed, blood may collect and form a clot. In addition to pain and redness, there may be considerable swelling around the site. The vein may also feel hard and cord-like, with evidence of warmth and redness and/or a red streak.

b. ***Intervention.*** Discontinue the infusion and start a new one in the opposite limb. Apply warm, moist compresses to the old site. Notify the physician. Chart your observations in the patient's record. NOTE: Suppurative thrombophlebitis—an extremely dangerous systemic complication—is described in section C-3. Because this complication can arise after an infusion has been discontinued, it is important to observe the patient carefully.

c. ***Suggestions for prevention***

> ➤ Check the site frequently for signs of soreness and/or redness.
> ➤ Infuse the medication at the prescribed rate of flow.
> ➤ Use the smallest-size catheter/needle that will meet the patient's needs and allow for adequate dilution in the vein.
> ➤ Dilute irritating medications with as much diluent as possible.
> ➤ Develop an atraumatic insertion technique.
> ➤ Tape the catheter/needle device securely to prevent unnecessary movement of the device in the vein.

6. Hematoma

a. ***What may happen.*** Blood may escape from the vein into the surrounding tissues or be infused into the tissues.

b. ***Intervention***

> ➤ If, during a transfusion, the blood is infused into the tissues, discontinue the infusion. Using a new venipuncture device, start the transfusion at another site, preferably in the opposite limb.
> ➤ If blood has escaped into the surrounding tissues because of a through-and-through penetration of the vein, remove the catheter/needle device and apply digital pressure to the site until the bleeding stops; if the bleeding appears to be severe and/or prolonged, cool compresses or an ice pack may be applied to the area.

> Once the possibility of continued bleeding into the tissues has ceased, warm, moist compresses may be applied to the limb to enhance the healing process.

C. SYSTEMIC PROBLEMS

1. Side effects, drug interactions, and adverse or allergic reactions

a. *What may happen.* The interaction or incompatibility of certain drugs, or the patient's sensitivity to a specific solution or medication may produce signs of adverse or allergic reactions. Some of these signs may include, but are not limited to:

> GI disturbances
> Central nervous system (CNS) depression
> Respiratory symptoms
> Anaphylaxis
> Rash/pruritus

These complications depend on the drug or drugs being given, on the dose and route of each, and on the individual patient. Obviously this book cannot cover such a large topic. You should, however, be aware of the common side effects, interactions, and adverse reactions that can occur with drugs that are given intravenously.

b. *Intervention*

> Slow the infusion to a KVO rate (if the symptoms are mild or questionable), or discontinue the infusion but keep the line open with 0.9% NaCI(NSS)
> Notify the patient's physician
> Chart your observations

c. *Suggestions for prevention*

> Check the patient's history of allergies before beginning an infusion

> ➤ Observe the patient frequently
> ➤ Administer the solution and/or medication according to the pharmacist's and the manufacturer's recommendations

2. Septicemia

a. ***What may happen.*** Bacteria or fungi may be introduced into an IV line at any point where one part is connected to another, particularly where the connection is performed manually. Poor design of IV equipment and improper manufacturing and storage have also been implicated in outbreaks of septicemia. Watch for these signs:

> ➤ Fever and/or chills
> ➤ Cold sweats
> ➤ Drop in blood pressure
> ➤ Nausea, vomiting, or diarrhea
> ➤ Increase in pulse rate

b. ***Intervention.*** Notify the physician. Consider other possible sites of origin for the septicemia (respiratory infection, urinary tract infection, wound infection, etc.) and culture any suspected sites. If no other sources of infection can be found, the IV system must be considered as the possible source—with or without signs of local infection. The IV site, tubing, bottle/bag, and any attachments should be cultured in accordance with your institution's policies, as outlined in Chapter 21. If the patient must continue to receive infusion therapy, another line may be started if necessary, but preferably in the opposite limb. Chart the procedure and your observations in the patient's record.

c. ***Suggestions for prevention***

> ➤ Always maintain aseptic technique
> ➤ Be careful not to contaminate the system when changing solutions, tubings, and dressings
> ➤ Keep all IV sites clean, dry, and covered with a sterile dressing

> Cleanse injection sites/adapters for 10-15 sec. prior to accessing

3. Suppurative thrombophlebitis

a. ***What may happen.*** The chain of events leading to this potentially fatal complication might start with irritation of the venous wall. Organisms enter the vein via contaminated IV solution, tubing, or insertion site. These organisms infect the irritated venous wall and a pocket of pus forms. This purulent thrombus then embolizes, releasing huge numbers of infective organisms into the patient's circulation and producing overwhelming sepsis.

b. ***Intervention.*** Unfortunately, signs of severe septicemia may be the first clinical warning of suppurative thrombophlebitis. Notify a physician and discontinue the infusion. The site, tubing, bottle/bag, and any attachments should be cultured in accordance with your institution's policies, as outlined in Chapter 21. Another line may be started, if necessary, in the opposite limb. Chart the procedure and your observations in the patient's record.

c. ***Suggestions for prevention***

> Always maintain aseptic technique
> Be careful not to contaminate the system when changing solutions, tubings, and dressings
> Keep all IV sites clean, dry, and covered with a sterile dressing.

4. Air embolism

a. ***What may happen.*** Air inadvertently introduced into the IV line may enter a vein. As little as 50 ml of air can cause an embolism in an adult; as little as 5 ml will do so in a small child. There is even a greater possibility that an air embolism will occur when dealing with a central line than when dealing with a peripheral line. An air embolism produces these symptoms:

> Drop in blood pressure
> Rapid, thready pulse
> Crushing chest pain
> Difficulty breathing, progressing to respiratory failure
> Cyanosis

b. Intervention

> Turn the patient on his or her left side and lower the head of the bed (Trendelenburg position).
> Try to determine the source of the air (e.g., disconnected line).
> Give the patient oxygen (2 to 3 liters) Notify the physician.
> Chart what you did and your observations in the patient's record.

c. Suggestions for prevention

> Make sure all connections on the IV line are securely fastened—Luer-Lok connections are highly recommended.
> Purge all air from the tubing before connecting the tubing to the patient.
> Change all tubings quickly, especially on central lines. You may have the patient forcibly exhale (Valsalva maneuver) when changing tubing on an open-end central line or close the clamp on the central line if one is present.

5. Catheter embolism

This is a greater possibility when inserting a CTN device than when using a CON device.

a. What may happen. A piece of catheter may be severed and may enter the circulatory system.
b. Intervention

➢ Discontinue the IV infusion.
➢ Apply a tourniquet to the patient's limb above the insertion site. Apply the tourniquet so that it is tight enough to restrict venous flow but not arterial flow.
➢ Notify the physician and have the patient x-rayed to locate the severed catheter.
➢ Chart what you did and your observations in the patient's record.

c. Suggestions for prevention

➢ Never reinsert the needle/stylet in the catheter once it has been withdrawn.
➢ Take special care when you withdraw a CTN device.
➢ When using scissors to remove an IV dressing, be extremely careful that the catheter is not accidentally cut.

6. Circulatory overload

a. What may happen. The patient may receive too much fluid for the circulatory system to handle. Circulatory overload produces these symptoms:

➢ Increase in blood pressure
➢ Distended veins in the neck, face, and arms
➢ Respirations become shallow and rapid (dyspnea)
➢ Rales may be detected
➢ Frothy sputum
➢ Productive cough

b. Intervention

➢ Slow the infusion to a KVO rate
➢ Elevate the head of the bed
➢ Apply oxygen (2 to 3 liters), provided it is not contraindicated
➢ Notify the patient's physician

➢ Chart what you did and your observations in the patient's record

c. *Suggestions for prevention*

➢ Monitor the patient's vital signs and intake and output carefully.
➢ Check the infusion flow rate regularly and notify the physician if it appears to be more than the patient can tolerate.
➢ Be aware of the patient's cardiovascular status and history before beginning the infusion.

CHAPTER 18

Blood Transfusions

Whole blood is not often administered. However, since administration of whole blood and some of its constituents—particularly packed red cells—creates unique problems, it is important to learn the rules and considerations that govern blood transfusions.

A. TERMINOLOGY

> **Agglutination:** The clumping of red cells by the formation of antibody bridges between antigens on different cells.
> **Antibody:** Protein in plasma that may react with a specific antigen.
> **Antigen:** A substance that has the ability to evoke an immune response when injected into an individual to whom it is foreign.
> **Bacteriolysin:** An antibody produced within the body that is capable of bringing about the dissolution or lysis of bacteria.
> **HLA:** Human leukocyte antigen.
> **Immunoglobulins:** Proteins with known antibody activity.
> **Rb (Rhesus):** The presence or absence of red blood cell D antigen.
> **Titer:** The amount of antibody in a serum.

B. BLOOD COMPONENTS

1. Plasma

> ➤ Water
> ➤ Gases
> ➤ Protein (albumin, globulins, fibrinogen)
> ➤ Salts (chlorides, bicarbonates, sulfates, phosphates)
> ➤ Protective substances (antibodies, bacteriolysins)
> ➤ Waste (urea, creatinine)

2. Cells

> ➤ Red blood cells—erythrocytes
> ➤ White blood cells—leukocytes (basophils, eosinophils, neutrophils, lymphocytes, monocytes)
> ➤ Platelets

C. COMPATIBILITY

Never give whole blood or packed red cells unless you are certain of donor-recipient compatibility, except in an extreme emergency on the orders of a physician. Type 0 blood may be administered in controlled situations (e.g., ER, OR, trauma unit) when dealing with life-and-death situations. Transfusion of a wrong blood type is prevented by crossmatching the donor's blood with the recipient's blood prior to initiation of the transfusion. Blood types are differentiated by their antigen and antibody content (see Table 18-1).

1. Requirements for different components

Blood is frequently utilized in component parts. Various components are indicated in specific circumstances. Not all of these components require typing and crossmatching. For those that do, however, the compatibility requirement is absolute, except as noted above. Table 18-2 is a guide to the infusion of blood and its various components.

Table 18-1.
Antigen and antibody content of various blood types

Blood type	Antigen type (found in RBC's)	Antibody type (found in plasma)
A	A	Anti-B
B	B	Anti-A
AB	A and B	None
O	None	Anti-A and anti-B

2. Safety

You may have the right blood, but the wrong recipient. A mistake like that could have disastrous—even fatal—results. Thus, the importance of safety cannot be over-stressed. To help prevent mistakes, the following steps are strongly recommended:

➢ Check the physician's order for the transfusion. If the patient is conscious, ask his/her name.

➢ Check the patient's name, birth date, and hospital identification number on the patient's ID bracelet with the label on the blood product.

➢ Have a second person recheck the above information.

➢ Take the patient's vital signs; if they are not within normal limits for that patient, notify the physician before initiating the transfusion.

➢ Be sure you have a patent line with an appropriate catheter/needle device. Normal (0.9%) saline is the only acceptable solution that may immediately precede or flush a blood infusion line.

➢ Record the procedure, and the number of the blood product infusing, in the patient's record.

➢ Monitor the patient's vital signs throughout the infusion (q15 mm x 2, then q30 mm until the procedure is finished). Monitoring schedules may be different according to your facilities' policies and procedures.

Table 18-2. Component therapy

Product	Indications for use	Average Infusion Time	Cross-matching
Whole blood	Increase blood volume ▸ Hemorrhage ▸ Trauma	2-4 hr	ABO and Rh
Packed red blood cells	Increase red cell mass ▸ Anemia	2-3 hr	ABO and Rh
Washed red blood cells	Increase red cell mass; prevent tissue antigen formation ▸ Immunosuppressed patients ▸ Patients with previous transfusion reactions	1-2 hr	ABO and Rh
White blood cells (leukophoresis)	Agranulocytosis	60-90 min	ABO and HLA (Preferably leuko-cyte group A antigen)
Fresh frozen plasma (FFP); 30-45 min for thawing	Coagulation disorders hypovolemia ▸ Burn patients	15-45 min	None
Platelets	Thrombocytopenia ▸ Leukemia patients ▸ Patients receiving massive transfusions	30-45 min for drip infusion; 5-10 min. for IV push	ABO
Cryoprecipitate (factor VIII)	Bleeding disorder due to lack of factor VIII; fibrinogen deficiency. ▸ Hemophilia ▸ Von Willebrand's disease	15-30 min for drip infusion; 5-10 min for IV push	ABO
Factor II, VII, IV, X complex	Bleeding disorder due to lack of these factors. ▸ Christmas Disease	15–30 min	None
Albumin, 5% or 25%	Blood volume expansion replacement of protein ▸ Burn patients ▸ Hypoproteinemia	30–60 min	None
Plasma protein fraction	Blood volume expansion; replacement of protein ▸ Hypovolemia ▸ Hypoproteinemia	30-60 min	None

D. EQUIPMENT FOR ADMINISTERING WHOLE BLOOD, PACKED RED CELLS, AND WASHED RED CELLS

1. Catheter/needle for venipuncture

   a. **Whole blood and washed red cells.** Use an 18-, 20-, or 22-gauge catheter: the largest size permitted by the patient's venous system and physical condition. For transfusion through a scalp vein, needles as small as 25 gauge may be used.

   b. **Packed red cells.** An 18-gauge catheter is best, but you may use a 20-gauge device for venipuncture if necessary.

2. Normal (0.9%) saline

In some institutions, it is customary to precede and follow transfusions of whole blood or blood components with normal saline. If normal saline is not already running, you may use a 250- or 500-ml bag of normal saline solution.

3. Straight-line blood set

This may be either a primary or secondary set. The drip chamber contains a filter, so you do not have to add a filter to the line. Use a large (16- or 18-gauge) needle to infuse the blood or packed cells into the primary line if the blood is a secondary set and a needless system is not being used. If the primary solution is not normal saline, you will have to replace it with normal saline. A straight-line set is also used for administering plasma, white cells, plasma protein fraction, and factors II, VII, IX, and X complex. The blood set should be changed after the infusion of two units.

4. Y-blood set

A Y-set may also be either a primary or secondary set. It is especially useful when the primary solution is not normal saline, as you do not have to replace the primary solution. A Y-set is advantageous for transfusion of packed red cells because it enables you to dilute the viscous cells with saline if necessary. Like a straight-line set, a

Y-set contains a filter in the drip chamber (see Figure 18-1). Attach the saline to one arm of the Y-set and the unit of blood to the other. To keep blood from backing up into the primary line, if you are piggybacking the Y-blood set into the primary set, close the clamp on the primary set. The Y-set should be changed after the infusion of two units of blood.

5. Microaggregate recipient set and filters

a. A microaggregate recipient set is used to transfuse large amounts—more than three units—of blood for immunosuppressed patients or for those with potential febrile leukocyte reactions. The special filter prevents lysed cells from reaching the patient's circulation, and the large tubing permits rapid administration. A micro-aggregate set may be used as a primary or secondary set.

b. Microaggregate add-on filters are added to straight IV tubing when three or more units of blood are to be infused over a short period of time. They function exactly the same way as microaggregate recipient sets except that the filter is separate and must be added to the IV tubing. Frequently used microaggregate filters are Bentley, Pall, Fenwal, and Swank.

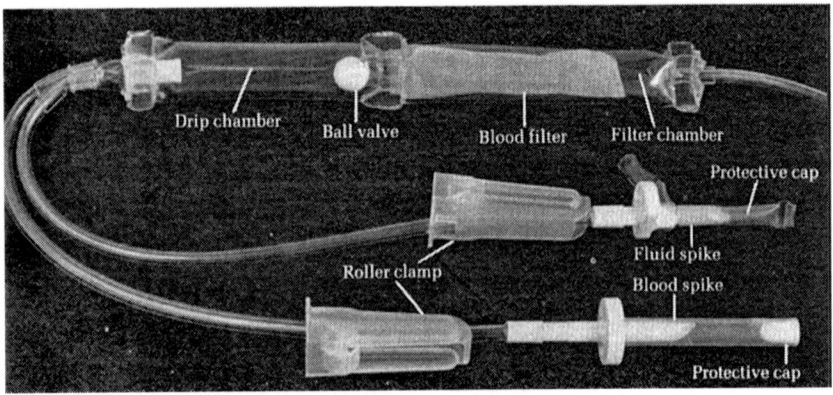

Figure 18-1. Y-blood tubing

6. Blood warmers

Never give large amounts of cold blood rapidly; that is likely to cause venous spasms and/or shock. Blood warmers should be used for patients receiving multiple units of blood, for those receiving blood through a central line, and for those who have cold agglutinins present in their blood.

   a. Coil type. Prime the coil, then close all clamps. Immerse the filled coil in water warmed to 99°F (37.6°C), taking care to keep both adapters dry.

   b. Electric type. After putting the blood-warming bag in the warmer and closing the door, let the warmer heat to 99°F. Prime the line with saline and start the transfusion according to the manufacturer's directions.

7. Transfusion pumps

Pumps are used to administer large amounts of blood quickly. They are not used routinely, and should be operated only by qualified personnel. Both types described here are operated by manual pressure. If you are using a very small catheter/needle, pumping can mechanically lyse red cells.

   a. Built-in type. This is a complete primary or secondary administration set, primed like any other. Make sure the pump chamber is completely filled before you squeeze it.

   b. Slip-on type. This pump may be used with a straight-line or Y-type set. After priming the set, slip the pump bag over the blood bag and hang both together. Open the screw clamp and squeeze the bulb until the gauge shows the desired pressure reading. Do not make the pressure so great that the needle on the pressure gauge goes into the red (danger) area.

E. EQUIPMENT FOR ADMINISTERING CRYOPRECIPITATE AND PLATELETS

1. Catheter/needle for venipuncture

An 18-gauge catheter is best, but a 20-gauge device may be used for venipuncture if necessary.

2. Component syringe set

A component syringe set is a secondary set. It permits rapid infusion of platelets—an important feature, since slow administration is likely to clog the primary line. The spiked (clamped) arm of this Y-shaped set is attached to the component bag; the other arm is connected to a 50- or 60-ml syringe. With the lower clamp closed, fill the syringe. Then close the upper clamp, open the lower one, and administer the component at the prescribed rate by IV push.

3. Component drip set

A component drip set can be used as either a secondary or a primary set.

F. CARE AND HANDLING OF BLOOD

1. Contamination

Blood and blood components are precious. They are also especially fertile breeding grounds for microorganisms. Take extra care to avoid inadvertent contamination when performing a transfusion.

2. Mixing whole blood

Red cells tend to settle and plasma tends to rise, so mix whole blood thoroughly. Avoid excessive agitation, though, as it may destroy cells. Gently rock the bag during transfusion to keep the red cells and plasma mixed.

3. Rate of administration

Federal regulations require that whole blood or packed red cells be transfused at rates no slower than one unit in four hours. Washed, packed, or fresh frozen red cells may be infused for between one and two hours, but no longer than four hours. Transfusions faster than one unit per hour should only be done if the patient's condition can tolerate it and in extreme emergencies under carefully controlled conditions.

G. MONITORING TRANSFUSIONS

Transfusion reactions may occur during, immediately after, or up to 96 hours following the transfusion.

1. Vital signs

Record vital signs just before and after each transfusion. During a transfusion, record vital signs every 15 minutes for the first half hour, and then every half hour until the transfusion is completed, or according to your institution's policy.

2. Hemolytic reactions

a Cause. Hemolytic reactions are due to separation of hemoglobin from either the recipient's or the donor's red cells during or following a transfusion. Hemolysis may be caused by any of several factors:

➤ Blood group incompatibility
➤ Rh incompatibility
➤ Injection of water or non-isotonic solutions

b. Severity. The severity of a hemolytic reaction depends on:

➤ The degree of ABO or Rh incompatibility
➤ The amount of blood administered

➢ The rate of administration
➢ The condition of the patient's liver, kidneys, and heart
➢ The temperature of the blood

c. **Symptoms**. If the patient complains of any of these symptoms, first try to rule out other causes, such as a history of emphysema, recovery from surgery under a general anesthetic, or the temperature of the room.

➢ Generalized tingling sensation
➢ Increased discomfort or anxiety
➢ Difficulty breathing
➢ Precordial pressure
➢ Bursting sensation in the head that is not due to anesthesia—a frequent cause of headache
➢ Flushed face
➢ Temperature elevation of more than 2°F
➢ Chills not due to hypothermia caused by anesthesia
➢ Severe pain in the neck, chest, or lumbar area that is not due to positioning during surgery or to pre-existing conditions

d. **Intervention**

➢ Check once more the patient's ID and blood numbers
➢ Clamp off the blood line, if it is still running, and administer normal saline
➢ Notify the physician and the laboratory
➢ Obtain required blood and urine samples
➢ Wait for the results of laboratory tests: If positive, disconnect the transfusion set, send it and the remaining blood to the lab, and notify the physician; if negative, slowly restart the transfusion and carefully observe the patient

e. **Prevention**

➢ Double-check the patient's name, identification number, and blood type before initiating transfusion

> ➢ Monitor the patient closely during the transfusion, especially during the first 30 minutes

3. Pyrogenic reactions

a. ***Cause.*** Pyrogenic reactions following transfusions are systemic reactions due to leukocyte agglutination or the presence of bacterial lipopolysaccharides.

b. ***Symptoms.*** First rule out other causes for the following symptoms:

> ➢ Chills
> ➢ Temperature elevation of more than 2°F
> ➢ Pain in the extremities or back

c. ***Intervention.*** Take the same steps as outlined for hemolytic reactions.

d. ***Prevention***

> ➢ An antipyretic medication may be administered prior to initiating the transfusion
> ➢ If the patient has had a previous reaction, washed or fresh frozen packed red cells should be used
> ➢ Keep the patient covered and warm during the transfusion
> ➢ Use a microaggregate blood filter

4. Allergic reactions

a. ***Cause.*** Allergic reactions are caused by hypersensitivity to some component of the donor's blood.

b. ***Symptoms.*** First rule out other causes for the following symptoms:

> ➢ Urticaria and pruritus
> ➢ Edema
> ➢ Dizziness and/or headache
> ➢ Nausea

> ➤ Chills (may be accompanied by a temperature elevation)
> ➤ Wheezing or dyspnea
> ➤ Lumbar pain

c. ***Intervention.*** Take the same steps as outlined for hemolytic reactions.

d. ***Prevention***

> ➤ If the patient has had a previous reaction, washed or fresh frozen packed red cells should be used
> ➤ An antihistamine (e.g., Benadryl) may be ordered prior to initiating the transfusion
> ➤ Monitor the patient closely during the transfusion, especially during the first 30 minutes

5. Circulatory overload

a. ***Cause.*** Circulatory overload may occur in the presence of heart disease with long-standing anemia. Circulatory overload may also occur when the cardiac musculature and reserve are deficient.

b. ***Symptoms.*** First rule out other causes for the following symptoms:

> ➤ Pulmonary congestion
> ➤ Signs of right-sided heart failure
> ➤ Dilated neck and arm veins
> ➤ Moist rales Flushed feeling
> ➤ Edema

c. ***Intervention.*** Take the same steps as outlined for hemolytic reactions.

d. ***Prevention***

> ➤ Use packed or washed red cells when the patient's cardiovascular system may be compromised
> ➤ Infuse the blood slowly
> ➤ Keep the patient warm and in a Fowler's position

> A diuretic may be ordered prior to initiating the transfusion
> Monitor the patient closely during the transfusion

6. Septicemia

a. *Cause.* Septicemia may be caused by infusion of contaminated blood or blood products, or by the presence of microorganisms somewhere within the transfusion line. Chapter 17 details the symptoms of septicemia.

b. *Intervention*

> Check once again the patient's ID and blood numbers
> Clamp off the blood line if it is still running, and hang a bag of normal saline
> Notify the physician
> Obtain required blood and urine samples
> Culture the puncture site, tubing, and bag in accordance with your institution's policy (see Chapter 21)
> Wait for the results of laboratory tests: if positive, disconnect the transfusion set, send it and the remaining blood to the lab, and notify the physician; if negative, slowly restart the transfusion and carefully observe the patient

c. *Prevention*

> Use strict aseptic technique when handling blood and blood products
> Avoid touch contamination of the infusion line
> Infuse the blood within the prescribed time
> Change the blood tubing after every one to two units

CHAPTER 19

Fluids And Electrolytes

We infuse many solutions and medications into our patients intravenously. These substances contain a variety of ingredients (electrolytes, vitamins, medications, etc.) and place a variety of demands on the body to adjust. Different disease processes, surgical procedures, and changes in physiology also produce a number of requirements and adjustments for the body to meet. If we are to be successful in restoring and maintaining the body in a state of homeostasis, and if we are to help our patients realize their optimal level of health and functioning, we must have a basic understanding of fluids and electrolytes, and learn to apply those principle in caring for our patients—Particularly those requiring intravenous therapy.

A. TERMINOLOGY

> *Anions:* Negatively charged ions.
> *Cations:* Positively charged ions.
> *Colloids:* Substances that do not dissolve in solution but form a gelatin-like substance.
> *Crenation:* An alteration of the external wall of a red blood cell due to a change in the internal fluid content.
> *Crystalloids:* Substances that completely dissolve to form a clear solution.
> *Diffusion:* Movement of solute molecules (gas, liquid, or solid) across a selectively permeable membrane from an area of high concentration to one of lower concentration.

- *Electrolytes:* Electrically charged particles (ions).
- *Extracellular:* Outside the cell.
- *Filtration:* The transfer of water and dissolved substances through a selectively permeable membrane from an area of high concentration to one of low concentration, based on hydrostatic pressure (mm Hg)—diffusion under pressure.
- *Hemolysis:* Movement of water from extracellular to intracellular space, which causes the red blood cell to swell and rupture.
- *Hypertonic:* Having a higher osmotic pressure than a compared solution.
- *Hypotonic:* Having a lower osmotic pressure than a compared solution.
- *Intracellular:* Inside the cell.
- *Isotonic:* A solution having a comparable concentration of solute particles that will exert an equivalent amount of osmotic pressure as that solution with which it is being compared.
- *Milliequivalent (mEq):* Measures the concentration of electrolytes in solution. Their chemical combining power is based on the number of available ionic charges in the solution.
- *Milliosmole (mOsm):* Measurement of osmotic activity in a given solution. The normal osmolality of body fluids is 280 to 294 mOsm/kg.
- *Osmosis:* Movement of water across a semipermeable membrane from the area of lower concentration to the area of higher concentration, thus tending to equalize the concentration of the two solutions.
- *Osmotic pressure:* The pressure that develops when two solutions of different concentrations are separated by a semipermeable membrane. Osmotic pressure varies with the concentration of the solution and the temperature variations.
- *Solutes:* Particles that are suspended or dissolved in a solvent.
- *Solution:* Made up of a solvent and solutes.
- *Solvent:* A liquid.
- *Tonicity:* The concentration of dissolved particles in solution as compared with plasma.

B. BODY FLUIDS

1. Water (H_2O)

   a. Amount. The amount of water contained in the body is dependent on:

- ➤ Age
- ➤ Weight
- ➤ Sex

   b. Body weight. The percentage of body weight accounted for by water is:

- ➤ Average male 60%
- ➤ Average female 54%
- ➤ Average infant 80%

2. Compartments

   a. Intracellular. This compartment accounts for approximately 40% of body weight.

   b. Extracellular

- ➤ Interstitial (surrounds the cell)—accounts for approximately 15% of body weight
- ➤ Intravascular (within the blood vessels)—accounts for approximately 5% of body weight

3. Electrolytes

In order to achieve chemical balance, the total number of positive charges must equal the total number of negative charges within each fluid compartment of the body.

- ➤ Principal extracellular electrolytes: Na^+, Ca^{2+}, Cl^-, HCO_3^-
- ➤ Principal intracellular electrolytes: K^+, Mg^{2+}, PO_4^{3-}

See the section on electrolytes below for a discussion of individual electrolytes.

4. Nonelectrolytes

a. Dextrose (D.Glucose)

➢ Normal serum level: 80 to 120 mg/dl
➢ Function: supplies necessary calories for energy (spares protein); converted to glycogen by the liver (improves hepatic function); daily requirement is approximately 100 grams per day.

b. Urea nitrogen

➢ Normal serum level: 10 to 20 mg/dl.

c. Creatinine

Normal serum level: 1 to 1.5 mg/dl.

C. ELECTROLYTES

1. Sodium (Na⁺)

Sodium is the principal extracellular cation.

➢ Normal serum level: 135 to 145 mEqL
➢ Function: regulates osmotic pressure of extracellular fluid and water balance within the body; also assists in the transmission of nerve impulses and influences the body's acid-base balance.

a. Hyponatremia

➢ Some causes: CHF; impaired renal function; cirrhosis; prolonged fever; diarrhea, vomiting, or gastric suctioning; burns; adrenal insufficiency; increased diaphoresis (a total day's sodium may be lost with 6 to 8 hours of diaphoresis)

➤ Signs and symptoms: muscle weakness; headache; decreased skin turgor; tremors and/or convulsions; serum sodium <135 mEq/L.

b. Hypernatremia

➤ Some causes: inadequate water intake; excess sodium intake; excessive water losses as in prolonged diarrhea; vomiting; polyuria; diabetes mellitus

➤ Signs and symptoms: thirst; dry, sticky membranes; fever; flushed skin, oliguria; serum sodium > 145 mEq/L.

2. Potassium (K^+)

Potassium is the principal intracellular cation.

➤ Normal serum level: 3.5 to 5.3 mEq/L
➤ Function: regulates cellular osmotic pressure; activates enzymes; regulates acid-base balance; assists with nerve impulse transmission in nerves and muscles

a. Hypokalemia

➤ Some causes: renal dysfunction; CHF; excessive use of diuretics; prolonged gastric suctioning; vomiting; diaphoresis or diarrhea; adrenal disorders; liver disease; starvation; ulcerative colitis; polyuria

➤ Signs and symptoms: decreased gastrointestinal, skeletal, and cardiac muscle function; decreased reflexes; muscular irritability or weakness; rapid, weak, and irregular pulse, decreased blood pressure; nausea and vomiting; paralytic ileus; ECG change; postural hypotension

b. Hyperkalemia

- ➤ Some causes: renal failure; massive cell damage, as in trauma, burns, major surgery, and myocardial infarction
- ➤ Signs and symptoms: muscle weakness; nausea; diarrhea; muscle irritability; oliguria; ECG changes

3. Calcium (Ca^{2+})

- ➤ Normal serum level: 8.5 to 10.5 mg/dl
- ➤ Function: important in formation and function of bones and teeth; aids in blood clotting; regulates neuromuscular excitability; assists in transfer of Na+ across semi-permeable membrane

a. Hypocalcemia

- ➤ Some causes: hypoparathyroidism; vitamin D or magnesium deficiency; pancreatitis; post-op thyroid or parathyroid patients; diarrhea; extensive infections; patients on prolonged TPN or dialysis; burns
- ➤ Signs and symptoms; muscle twitching and cramps; perioral paresthesia; carpopedal spasms; tetany; convulsion

b. Hypercalcemia

- ➤ Some causes: hyperparathyroidism; overdose of vitamin D or antacids; skeletal diseases; carcinomas (such a parathyroid adenoma and multiple myeloma)
- ➤ Signs and symptoms: lethargy; anorexia; nausea; vomiting; constipation; dehydration; cardiac arrhythmias; coma

4. Magnesium (Mg^{2+})

- ➤ Normal serum level: 1.5 to 2.5 mEq/L

➢ Function: controls action of enzymes; assists in metabolism of proteins and carbohydrates; aids in controlling neuromuscular irritability; facilitates transportation of Na+ and K+ across cell membranes.

a. Hypomagnesemia. This condition usually coexists with low Ca^{2+} and K^+ levels.

➢ Some causes: impaired gastrointestinal absorption; diarrhea; inadequate diet; hyperparathyroidism; excessive use of diuretics; prolonged vomiting or nasogastric suctioning; renal dysfunction; chronic alcoholism
➢ Signs and symptoms: cardiac arrhythmias; muscle weakness; seizures; tremors; tetany; cramps in the lower extremities; insomnia; disorientation

b. Hypermagnesemia

➢ Some causes: renal failure; excessive use of antacids
➢ Signs and symptoms: hypotension; flushing; sweating; slow, weak pulse; lethargy; decreased respirations; muscle weakness; decreased reflexes; coma; bradycardia; heart block; cardiac arrest

5. Chloride (Cl^-)

➢ Normal serum level: 95 to 109 mEq/L
➢ Function: Competes with bicarbonate for combination with Na^+ ions; assists in maintaining acid-base balance

a. Hypochloremia

➢ Some causes: prolonged nasogastric suctioning; excessive use of diuretics; prolonged diaphoresis, gastrointestinal suctioning; diabetic ketosis; CHF; renal failure—low-salt diet—metabolic alkalosis

➤ Signs and symptoms: increased muscle excitability; tetany; decreased respirations

b. Hyperchloremia

➤ Some causes: dehydration: hyperparathyroidism; metabolic acidosis; respiratory alkalosis
➤ Signs and symptoms: stupor; deep, rapid breathing; coma; muscle weakness

6. Phosphate (PO_4^{3-})

➤ Normal serum level: 1.7 to 2.3 mEq/L
➤ Function: assists with glucose metabolism in red cells; essential for ATP (adenosine triphosphate) formation; acts as a check and balance for Ca^{2+} (inverse relationship with calcium)

a. Hypophosphatemia

➤ Some causes: hyperparathyroidism; rickets; osteomalacia; abnormalities of the renal tubules
➤ Signs and symptoms: circumoral and peripheral paresthesia; lethargy; speech defects (stuttering or stammering)

b. Hyperphosphatemia

➤ Some causes: excessive growth hormone (acromegaly); hypoparathyroidism or pseudohypoparathyroidism; renal insufficiency or acute failure; hypervitaminosis D
➤ Signs and symptoms: usually none

7. Bicarbonate (HCO_3^-)

➤ Normal serum level: 24 to 32 mEq/L
➤ Function: chief buffer in maintaining acid-base balance (a deficit will cause metabolic acidosis

and an overabundance will result in metabolic alkalosis)

8. Proteinate

a. Albumin

> Normal serum level: 3.5 to 5.5.g/dl
> Function: assists with cell repair; healing of wounds; synthesis of vitamins and enzymes; moving substances from the interstitial fluid into the vascular system; maintaining colloidal osmotic pressure

b. Globulin

> Normal Serum level: 1.5 to 3g/dl
> Function: same as for albumin

9. Sulfate (SO_4^{2-})

> Normal serum level: 0.5 to 1.5 mg/dl
> Function: basic material of proteins; assists in maintaining acid-base balance

10. Carbonic acid

Carbonic acid may act as a cation or an anion

> Function: acts as a buffer in maintaining balance between the number of cations and anions in the body

11. Trace Elements

a. Cobalt

> Function: the principal constituent of vitamin B_{12}

b. Copper

> Function: essential in preventing anemia

c. Iodine

> Function: essential for thyroid function

d. Zinc

> Function: essential for wound healing and enzyme activity

e. Manganese

> Function: essential for skeletal growth, in addition to Ca^{2+} and phosphorus metabolism

D. VITAMINS

Vitamins are necessary for the utilization of nutrients and for physiological functions.

1. B andC

> Water soluble
> Important in metabolism of carbohydrates; promo healing: help maintain gastrointestinal function

2. A,D,E, and K

> Fat Soluble
> Important in bone formation, calcium and phosphorus absorption, and prothrombin formation
> Overingestion may cause hypervitaminosis

E. ACID-BASE BALANCE

The acid balance depends on the hydrogen ion concentration

1. Normal pH of blood

The normal range of pH in extracellular fluid is 7.35 to 7.45 (extreme limits compatible with life are 6.9 to 7.8)

2. Regulatory mechanisms

The body attempts to maintain its fluid and electrolyte balance through utilization of:

> ➤ Circulatory (cardiovascular) buffer system
> ➤ Respiratory system (lungs)
> ➤ Renal system (kidneys)
> ➤ Endocrine system (posterior pituitary, parathyroids, adrenals)

F. MONITORING PARAMETERS

A patient's fluid and electrolyte status requires careful monitoring.

1. Clinical monitoring measures

    a. **Central venous pressure**
    b. **Pulse.** Monitoring includes both quality and rate
    c. **Venous fill of peripheral veins.** The normal venous fill is 3 to 5 seconds
    d. **Weight.** A 5% change in body weight indicates a serious shift; 1 kilogram of body weight (2.2 pounds) reflects 1 liter of body fluid
    e. **Thirst.** This occurs with loss of 1 liter of body fluid
    f. **I&O (intake and output).** Output should equal 30 to 50 ml/hr
    g. **Skin turgor**
    h. **Edema**

> ➢ Generalized (e.g., CHF)
> ➢ Localized (e.g., ascites)
> ➢ Peripheral

2. Laboratory monitoring measures

a. *Electrolyte studies*
b. *Blood cell count and hematocrit.* These detect hemoconcentration or hemodilution
c. *BUN*
d. *Serum protein measurement with albumin-globulin ratio*

G. FLUID THERAPY

1. Quality of solution

Before initiating infusion, check solution for:

> ➢ Valid expiration date
> ➢ Clarity (no particles or cloudiness)

2. Tonicity of solution

Tonicity affects fluid and electrolyte balance.

a. *Hypertonic fluids.* Hypertonic fluids (e.g., 3% NaCl or 10%, 20%, 50% dextrose) increase the osmotic pressure of the blood plasma and draw fluid out of the cells, causing shrinkage of the red blood cells—crenation—if infused over a long period of time[*] (see Figure 19-1). Such fluids:

> ➢ Should be infused through large (central) veins to allow for rapid dilution

---

[*] New theory may disagree with this concept.

> May cause osmotic diuresis and cellular dehydration if infused rapidly or for an extended period of time

b. Hypotonic fluids. Hypotonic fluids (e.g., 2.5% dextrose, 0.2% and 0.45% NaCl) decrease the osmotic pressure of the blood plasma and draw fluid into the cells, resulting in rupture of the red blood cells—hemolysis—if infused over a long period of time (see Figure 19-2). Such fluids:

> May be infused through peripheral veins
> May produce water intoxication and cerebral edema if infused for an extended period of time

c. Isotonic fluids. Isotonic fluids (e.g., 5% dextrose, 0.9% NaCl, Lactated Ringer's) maintain the osmotic pressure of the blood plasma and increase the extra-cellular fluid volume. Such fluids:

> May be infused through peripheral veins
> May result in circulatory overload if infused over a prolonged period of time or too rapidly

3. Normal maintenance

a. Water

> Individual requirements based on age, weight, and sex
> Insensible losses equal approximately 1,000 to 1,500 milligram per day
> Additional losses through urine, feces, and vomitus
> Essential for all body functions—primary constituent of all body fluids
> Hypotonic—must be combined with NaCl or dextrose to be given intravenously

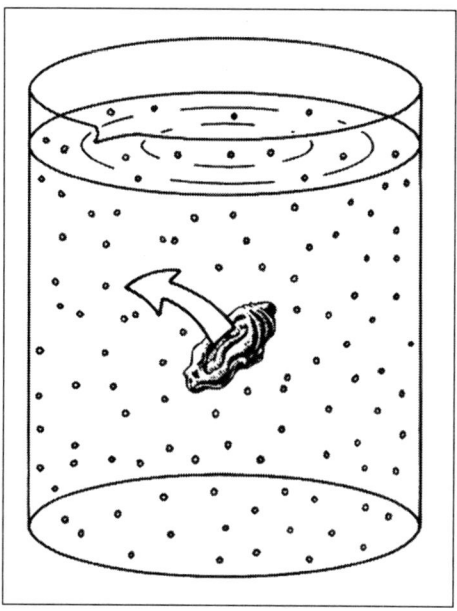

Figure 19-1. Crenation

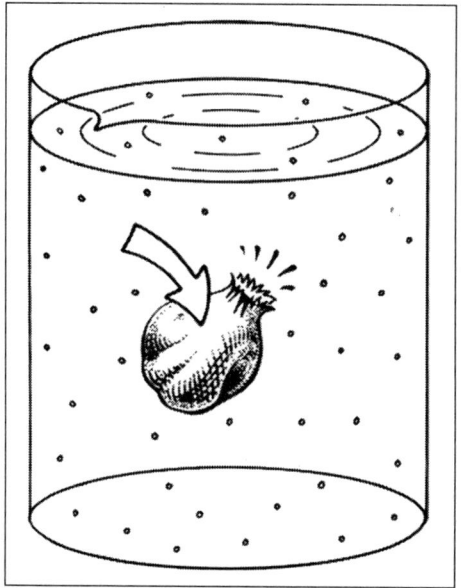

Figure 19-2. Hemolysis

b. *Glucose*

> ➤ Normal serum level: 80 to 120 mg/dl; maintained by action of insulin produced by the islets of Langerhans of the pancreas
> ➤ Daily requirement for the average adult: 100 grams per day
> ➤ Supplies necessary calories for energy—spares body protein
> ➤ Most important carbohydrate in body metabolism—excess glucose is converted to glycogen by the liver

c. *Protein*

> ➤ Daily requirement based on age, weight, daily activities, and state of health: average adult—1 gram per kilogram of body weight per day; average child—2 to 2.2 grams per kilogram of body weight per day
> ➤ Essential for growth, maintenance, and repair of body tissues
> ➤ Major source of heat and energy for the body

d. *Fats*

> ➤ Daily requirement for the average adult: 50 to 130 grams per day restricted intake for patients with hepatitis or those on low-calorie diets
> ➤ Important source of energy—spares body protein
> ➤ Provides essential fatty acids necessary for normal growth and development
> ➤ Serves as vehicle for absorption of fat-soluble vitamins

4. Replacement of losses

a. ***Maintain intake and output record.*** Adequate kidney function is critical when infusing large amounts of fluids and electrolytes.

b. ***Monitor patient.*** The body's need for fluid and electrolyte replacement increases when:

➢ The patient is febrile
➢ The patient is diaphoretic
➢ Cell trauma occurs (due to injury, surgery)
➢ Respirations are increased

c. ***Verify Type:*** Type of replacement depends on type of loss.

H. TYPES OF FLUID

We cannot possibly cover all the types of intravenous fluid available on the market, but the following are commonly used solutions.

1. Dextrose in Water

a. 5% (isotonic)

➢ Daily adult requirement: 1,500 to 2,500 ml per day
➢ Uses: solution for administration of intravenous medication; hydration (may cause circulatory overload, dilutional hyponatremia or hypokalemia, or water intoxication if infused over a prolonged period of time)

b. 10%, 20%, or 50% (hypertonic)

➢ Daily adult requirement: same as for 5%
➢ Uses: treatment of hyperkalemia (may cause dilutional hypokalemia or hyponatremia if infused over a prolonged period of time without electrolytes); to provide nutrition (insulin may need to be added to prevent overtaxing the pancreas)

2. Sodium chloride (NaCl)

a. Isotonic (0.9%)

➢ Uses: extracellular fluid replacement (may cause electrolyte imbalances if used exclusively for a prolonged period of time); flushing (TPN lines; before and after incompatible medications); initiating and terminating blood transfusions; treatment of metabolic alkalosis (overhydration may cause acidosis)

➤ May cause hyponatremia, circulatory overload, or hypokalemia if large amounts are infused for prolonged periods of time

b. Hypotonic (02% and 0.45% NaCl)

➤ Uses: as an electrolyte replenisher and for hydration

➤ May produce water intoxication and cerebral edema if infused over an extended period of time

c. Hypertonic (3% and 5% NaCl)

➤ Uses: replacement for severe sodium losses; treatment for dilutional hyponatremia and edema

➤ May produce cellular dehydration if infused over an extended period of time

3. Dextrose and sodium chloride combined

a. 5% dextrose with 0.9% NaCl ($D_5/0.9$)

➤ Uses: extracellular fluid replacement; prevent catabolism (formation of ketones) with loss of potassium and intracellular fluid

b. 2.5% or 5% dextrose together with 0.2% or 0.45% NaCl

➤ Uses: for hydration; to promote diuresis in dehydrated patients or to assess kidney function

4. Electrolyte solution (lactated Ringer's)

➤ Uses: extracellular fluid replacement (may produce circulatory overload if infused over a prolonged period of time); treatment of mild acidosis

➤ Contraindicated for patients with cardiac dysfunction or liver disease, or severe metabolic acidosis or alkalosis

CHAPTER 20

Parenteral Nutrition, Lipid Emulsions

Total parenteral nutrition (TPN)—also known as hyperalimentation—and lipid emulsion feeding are likely to be long-term regimens. Both TPN and lipid solutions are fertile breeding grounds for microorganisms. Therefore, extra care should be taken to observe strict aseptic technique in preparing, handling, and administering TPN and lipid solutions. TPN should be prepared under a laminar-flow hood by a trained Pharmacist using sterile technique.

A. *TOTAL PARENTERAL NUTRITION (TPN)*

1. Definition

TPN is the intravenous administration of carbohydrates, protein and fat to maintain protein anabolism and tissue synthesis.

2. Indications for use

 a. *Patients with pathological conditions necessitating high caloric and protein requirements.* Such patients would include those with:

  - Burns
  - Multiple systems trauma
  - Acute renal failure
  - Ulcerative colitis

- Crohn's disease
- Postoperative debilitation.

b. Patients unable to ingest food. Such patients would include those with:

- Crohn's disease with obstruction
- Esophageal or gastric carcinoma with upper G.I. obstruction
- Paralytic ileus

c. Patients who refuse to eat. They include:

- Psychiatric patients with depression or anorexia nervosa
- Geriatric patients

d. Patients who are unable to ingest sufficient calories or metabolize their food adequately to maintain a healthy nutritional status:

- Patients with AIDS
- Ulcerative colitis
- Wasting syndrome

3. Duration of therapy

Duration of TPN is totally dependent on the individual patient's overall condition, and the extent and nature of injury or disease. TPN may be given over a short period of time (7 to 10 days) or therapy may extend for a period of several months or years.

4. Type of line

TPN must be administered through a central vein. Any of the central lines are appropriate for the administration of TPN:

a. Percutaneously inserted non-tunneled central line (CVC)—frequently located in the subclavian, jugular or femoral.

b. **Tunneled catheters:** Open-end or Closed-end
c. **PORT's**
d. **PICC lines**

NOTE: A central line insertion is regarded as a major procedure performed by a physician (specially trained RN's may insert PICC lines). Placement of the central line must be confirmed by x-ray to insure correct catheter location (superior vena cava) before TPN therapy can be initiated. To keep the vein open until the x-ray can be done and the TPN started, a standard Isotonic IV solution—normal saline (0.9% NaCl) or 5% Dextrose in water (D5/W)—may be infused.

5. Starting the TPN

After the catheter's position has been verified by x-ray, you should be ready to start the TPN infusion. The solution should be kept at room temperature for one hour prior to infusing; cold fluids infused directly from the refrigerator may cause a serious venospasm.

- Remove the protective cap from the TPN bottle and wipe the stopper with an alcohol wipe or remove the tab from the bag
- Take down the 5% dextrose or normal saline solution, hung to maintain the line, clamp off the tubing, and pull out the tubing spike from the IV bag
- Insert the tubing spike into the TPN bottle/bag and prime the tubing
- Connect the tubing to the pump and set the desired flow rate
- Open the clamp on the IV tubing and start the pump

6. Monitoring the patient

a. **Complications of TPN.** Because of the danger of contamination, the invasiveness of the catheter, the high glucose concentration, the electrolyte composition of the TPN solution, and the large amounts infused, many serious complications are possible. Additional complications may be introduced by the practice of giving supplemental insulin to process the large amounts of glucose in the TPN solution. Therefore, it's essential to observe the patient for developments of possible complications such as:

- Blood glucose over 200 mg/dl : hyperglycemia
- Urine glucose over 1+ : hyperglycemia or osmotic diuresis
- Rapid pulse, increased blood pressure, diaphoresis : hypoglycemia
- Elevated temperature, redness, pain, exudate from the catheter exit site : infection (catheter associated septicemia should always be considered in the differential diagnosis of fever)
- Swelling around the insertion site, face or neck : infiltration, venous thrombosis or formation of a fibrin sheath/flap
- Edema, weakness, restlessness, rapid breathing, pallor, flushing, cramps, headache, nausea: electrolyte or acid-base imbalance
- Distended veins in neck, arm, and hands, elevated blood pressure : fluid overload
- Increased BUN (negative nitrogen balance): hyperglycemic, hyperosmotic nonketotic acidosis (inadequate caloric intake resulting in protein catabolism).
- Weight loss : inadequate TPN (under nutrition)
- Labored breathing, pain/pressure in the chest : air embolism

b. **Documentation.** Follow your facility's policy in recording the following observations in the patient's chart:

- Vital signs—eight hours to once a day initially
- Urinary sugar, acetone, and specific gravity—every eight hours to once a day initially (use Clinistix or Testape, not Clinitest, if the patient is on an antibiotic)
- Body weight—weekly
- Fluid intake and output—initially daily

- Electrolytes, BUN, creatinine, triglycerides, cholesterol and other specified blood work—once or twice a week initially
- Blood sugar—initially daily

Once a patient has stabilized out on their TPN solution, the monitoring data can be reduced to once a week, once or twice a month or longer.

7. Dressing and tubing changes

a. Frequency: Change the dressing three times a week if a gauze dressing is utilized. If a transparent dressing is utilized the dressing change may be done once a week and prn. Transparent dressings should not be placed over the top of gauze dressings. The catheter sites should always be kept clean and dry. Replace the administration set every 24 hours. A 0.22 micron filter should be used on all plain TPN infusions (if lipids have been added to the TPN solution—then either a lipid filter, (1.2 micron), or no filter should be used). A filter less than 1.2 microns used on lipids will filter out the lipid emulsion. The tubing and filter are changed daily to safeguard against sepsis due to possible proliferation of microorganisms within the system.

b. Procedure. Procedure for dressing and tubing changes is essentially the same as for the initial setup and dressing. When you remove the dressing, carefully inspect the site and surrounding skin for exudate from the catheter exit site, redness, swelling and general condition. Examine the old dressing for evidence of blood, pus, or TPN solution.

c. Precautions

- Use sterile, no-touch technique, don mask and sterile gloves
- Make the change at the catheter-tubing junction as quickly as possible
- If the patient is on a respirator, and has a percutaneously inserted CVC, perform the tubing change on the expiratory cycle to help prevent a possible air embolism

- Ask the patient to turn his/her head in the opposite direction of the site during the procedure to help prevent contamination of the site

8. Additional precautions

- Keep the dressing clean and dry
- Keep the flow rate constant (less than 10% change per hour is recommended). If the rate is increased too rapidly to "catch up," it may throw the patient into hyperglycemia or osmotic diuresis: if the rate is decreased too rapidly, it could throw the patient into hypoglycemia.
- Never discontinue TPN therapy abruptly. The rapid decrease in the patient's blood sugar may cause hypoglycemia. Wean the patient down slowly over a couple of hours, especially if the TPN solution has a high dextrose content (30%-50%). If the TPN solution is inadvertently discontinued, a 10% dextrose solution may be hung in the interim until the patient's system can adjust and the infusion discontinued.
- Don't routinely draw blood through the TPN catheter; use another lumen on the catheter or a different route if necessary (eg. Peripheral stick).
- Don't piggyback any medication or solution through a TPN line.◻

9. Other considerations

- It is very important for the patient to maintain good oral hygiene.
- The psychological aspect of not eating in the "normal" fashion can be devastating to a patient. Support groups or counseling may be indicated to assist in adjusting to long term TPN.

◻   *The guidelines issued by the Centers for Disease Control state: "In an effort to avoid unnecessary contamination, the hyperalimentation system should not be used to measure the central venous pressure, administer blood products or 'piggyback' medications, or obtain blood samples." However, some institutions follow more liberal policies.*

B. LIPID EMULSIONS

Lipid emulsions are considered isotonic and therefore may be infused either peripherally or through a central line. They may be administered alone or added to a TPN or Amino Acid solution or piggybacked into the TPN line. Because lipid emulsions are a colloidal suspension, they should:

- never be delivered through a filter with a micropore size smaller than 1.2
- never be shaken vigorously
- be infused through a catheter/needle size of 20ga or larger

1. Purpose

Lipid emulsions may be given:

- To meet basic caloric needs. Approximately 2 bottles (1,000ml) of 10% lipids are required on a weekly basis to maintain basic metabolic requirements.
- To augment TPN therapy and provide additional calories when needed without appreciably increasing the total fluid volume.
- To help prevent fatty acid deficiencies.
- To increase general nutritional status and assist with the absorption of fat-soluble vitamins (A, D, E, K).

2. Contraindications

Lipid emulsions may be contraindicated for patients who suffer from:

- Severe hepatic or pulmonary disease
- A bone marrow dyscrasia
- A blood coagulation defect caused by a decreased platelet count
- Hyperlipemia

3. Equipment

- Bottle of lipid emulsion (500ml of 10% or 20%)

- Vented tubing
- Alcohol wipes
- Syringe with 5-10ml NSS flush
- Tape

4. Procedure

All lipid emulsion is generally administered through a primary line (it may be added directly to the TPN solution to form a 3-in-1 mixture).

- Lipids do not need to be refrigerated. However, if the solution was in the refrigerator, it should be allowed to stand at room temperature for at least 60 minutes before infusing.
- Examine the bottle for inconsistencies of color or texture (don't shake the bottle)
- Wipe the stopper of the bottle with alcohol
- Close the regulator clamp on the IV administration set
- Insert the spike into the stopper on the top of the Lipid bottle
- Prime the tubing
- Wipe the prn adapter injection site on the hub of the catheter (10-15 seconds)
- Remove the cap from the distal end of the IV tubing and attach the tubing to the prn adapter injection port
- Regulate the flow rate

If the lipid emulsion is to be utilized as a piggyback infusion:

- Examine the bottle for inconsistencies of color or texture (don't shake the bottle)
- Wipe the stopper of the bottle with alcohol
- Close the regulator clamp on the IV administration set
- Insert the spike into the stopper on the top of the Lipid bottle
- Prime the tubing
- Hang the bottle of lipid emulsion on the IV pole
- Wipe the needless adapter on the primary IV lubing (10-15 seconds)
- Attach the lipid tubing to the needless adapter port on the TPN tubing

- Be sure there are no filters in the lipid line or that the filter is a 1.2 lipid filter. If the primary TPN solution has a 0.22 micron filter in the tubing be sure to hang the lipid emulsion below the filter in the TPN line.
- Regulate the rate of flow

Regardless of the method of administration, lipid emulsions should always be started slowly and the patient observed closely for possible reactions, particularly in the first 30 minutes. If no reactions are noted, the rate may be increased. Be sure to:

- Label the bottle and tubing appropriately
- Chart the procedure and any pertinent observations in the patient's record
- Never add any fluid or medications to the lipid emulsion

5. Monitoring the patient

a. Complications of lipid-emulsion feeding.

Infusion at too fast a rate can cause fatty acid overload. The rate of administration should not exceed 500 ml in four hours. Patients may also experience adverse reactions to the lipid emulsion itself. Immediate signs of an adverse reaction include:

- Elevated temperature
- Flushing, sweating
- Nausea and vomiting
- Headache
- Chest and back pains
- Labored breathing

A patient who tolerates a lipid emulsion over a short period may still develop complications over several days' duration:

- Enlarged liver, jaundice
- Enlarged spleen, bleeding

- Focal seizures
- Peptic ulcer
- Hyperlipemia
- Thrombocytopenia

b. *Documentation.* Follow your facility's policy in recording the following observations in the patient's record:

- Vital signs (temperature, pulse, respirations and blood pressure)
- Fluid intake and output
- Body weight
- Caloric intake
- Serum turbidity (fatty acid clearance), triglycerides and cholesterol
- Hepatic function tests for patients receiving lipid emulsions for prolonged periods of time
- Other studies as ordered

6. Changing bottles and tubing

a. *Frequency.* Use a new tubing every time you hang a new bottle of lipid emulsion. If you're not going to give another bottle right away, remove the catheter/needle or convert the site to a heparin or saline lock. If you're going to start another bottle immediately, simply connect the new tubing to the hub of the catheter/needle after the tubing has been primed. Discard any remaining emulsion in the discontinued line.

b. *Procedure.* The procedure for intermittent infusion is the same as that for starting an infusion, except that you would connect the line to the PRN adapter (heparin/saline).

C. *PERIPHERAL PARENTERAL NUTRITION (PPN)*

Peripheral parenteral nutrition (PPN) is the peripheral administration of amino acids with electrolytes and sometimes with vitamins and mineral additives. These solutions may be administered alone or in conjunction with dextrose (not to exceed 10% when given peripherally) and lipid emulsions.

D. PROTEIN SUPPLEMENTATION

Some patients may need to have additional protein administered intravenously for a limited period of time. These patients include those:

- with low protein serum levels
- with draining wounds that are difficult to heal (especially stage III & IV)
- with poor nutritional status
- who are unable to take PO for short periods of time (2-4 weeks where you don't want them to loose additional nutritional ground

1. Purpose

PPN provides nutritional support for patients with little or no oral intake for periods of short duration (usually 2-8 weeks)or where a loss in nutritional status is of concern. For prolonged periods of inadequate nutritional intake, TPN should be considered. Patients receiving PPN should not anticipate a significant increase in their nutritional needs for any extended period of time.

2. Equipment

- Bottle of PPN solution
- Tubing
- Alcohol wipe

3. Procedure

The procedure for administering a PPN solution is the same as that for administering any primary solution (see Chapters 8 and 9).

4. Monitoring the patient

The patient's nutritional and hydration status should be assessed frequently to assure that the solutions being delivered are adequate to meet his/her needs. Serum glucose, electrolytes, BUN, and creatinine levels should be checked periodically to assist in verifying the patient's status.

CHAPTER 21

Infection Control In IV Therapy

The preceding chapters have mentioned, in an incidental way, the practical steps necessary to avoid infection. This chapter summarizes the ways in which IV systems can become contaminated with microorganisms and suggests measures for preventing infections resulting from IV therapy.

A. SOURCES OF INFECTION

1. Intrinsic and extrinsic

a. *Intrinsic.* Intrinsic sources of contamination are those present in the IV equipment before unpackaging and use:

- Cracks in bottles
- Punctures in bags
- Contaminated solution or blood
- Administration set contamination
- Venipuncture device contamination
- Ointments
- Gauze, tape, etc. used for dressings

b. Extrinsic. Extrinsic sources of contamination are those introduced in setting up and running an infusion:

- Additives
- Attachment of the bottle/bag to the administration set
- Infusion pump/volume controller or volume-control chamber
- Piggybacks
- Secondary infusions
- Add-on-filter
- Insertion of catheter/needle
- Stopcocks
- CVP manometer
- Flushing the line
- Injections into the line
- Inadequate cleansing of adapters prior to accessing the line

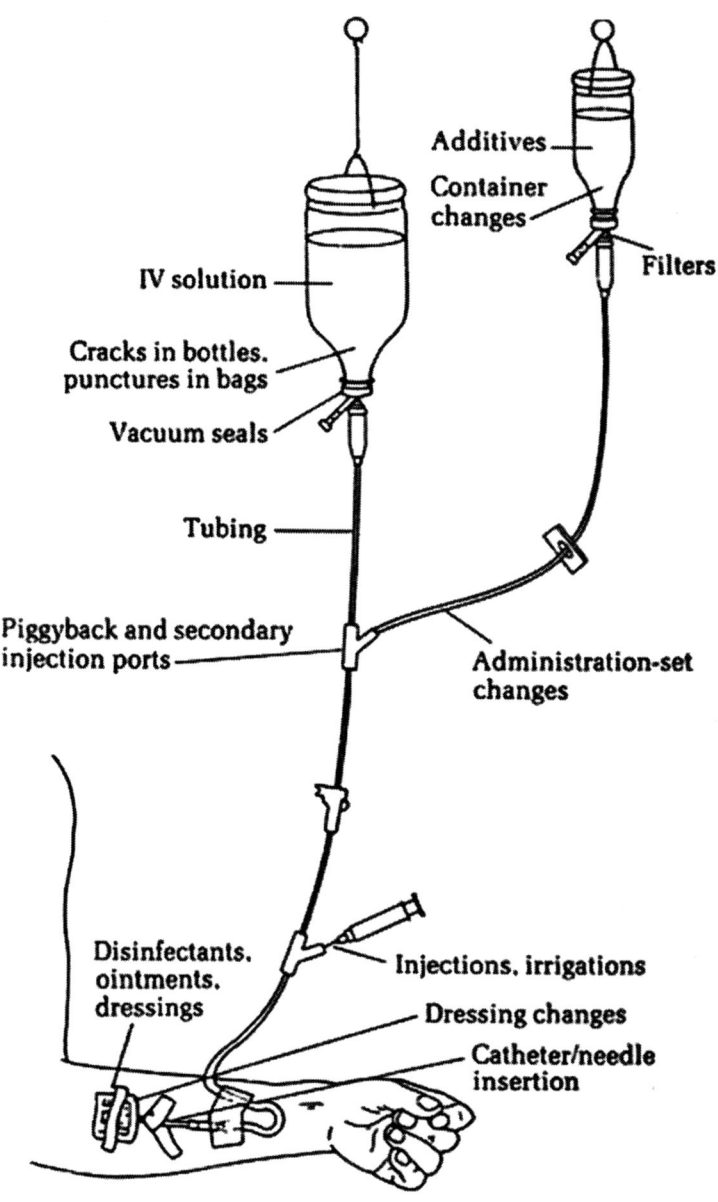

Additives
Container changes
Filters
IV solution
Cracks in bottles, punctures in bags
Vacuum seals
Tubing
Piggyback and secondary injection ports
Administration-set changes
Disinfectants, ointments, dressings
Injections, irrigations
Dressing changes
Catheter/needle insertion

The illustration (**Figure 21-1**) summarizes intrinsic and extrinsic sources of contamination.

2. Patient's skin flora

a. *Organisms*. The organisms that are most commonly cultured from catheter tips are Staphylococcus epidermidis, Staphylococcus aureus, Bacillus, Corynebacterium, Pseudomonas aeruginosa, Acinetobacteria species, Candida, gram-negative Bacilli and Enterococcus. A similar microbial profile has been observed in cases of catheter-associated septicemia. All these organisms are normal skin and body flora and therefore should be expected to be present on hospitalized patients and staff.

b. *Mechanisms of contamination*. It's been suggested that skin flora gain access to catheter tips in several ways:

- At the moment of insertion (touching the site after it has been prepped)
- By migrating along the interface between the catheter and the patient's tissues (if IV sites are not kept clean and dry)
- By insufficient cleansing of prn adapters and IV tubing injection ports prior to accessing (prior to accessing an IV injection port or prn adapter it should be firmly cleansed with an alcohol wipe for 10-15 seconds)

c. *Prevention*

- Thorough adequate cleansing of the patient's skin
- Immobilization of catheters/needles in the patient's vein
- Maintaining the site clean and dry
- Cleansing the injection ports, prn adapters, adequately prior to accessing

3. Health care Personnel

a. *Organisms*. In addition to the organisms normally present on skin, antibiotic-resistant gram-negative bacteria frequently contaminate the hands of healthcare personnel.

b. *Mechanisms of contamination*

- Failure to wash hands sufficiently
- Touching the IV site after it has been prepped
- Not prepping adequately
- Not allowing the prep solution to dry prior to sticking for a peripheral line
- Touching portions of IV equipment that should not be touched (i.e., needle and catheter tips, tubing ends, stoppers on bottles/bags
- Unnecessary manipulation of IV systems that are running
- Not cleansing access ports on IV tubings and PRN adapters sufficiently prior to accessing. Studies have shown that access devices should be cleansed with alcohol for a minimum of 10-15 seconds prior to accessing the IV line
- Not maintaining the IV dressing occlusive, clean and dry
- Insufficient flushing of the IV line that allows blood to remain in the line or prn adapter device (this promotes the growth of bacteria)

c. *Prevention*

- Wash hands vigorously with antimicrobial soap before initiating an infusion, before manipulating the system (i.e., tubing changes), and between patients
- Always avoid touch contamination
- Do NOT touch the site after it has been prepped (even with gloves on your hands)
- Don't handle any component of an IV system more than is necessary
- Cleanse the access devices (prn adapters) for 10-15 seconds with alcohol prior to accessing the line
- Keep all IV sites clean, occlusive and dry
- Flush lines sufficiently to remove all blood from the line, injection ports and prn adapters

4. Hospital environment

Hospital air, surfaces, and fomites are generally considered not to be a significant sources of microbial infection. However, don't expose any portion of an IV system to the air longer than is necessary, and be careful not to let any sterile portion of the system touch a non-sterile surface. Keep all ports on stopcocks covered at all times: stopcocks are a major source of contamination of IV systems. Keep all IV systems as "closed" as possible.

5. The patient

It's been found that the rate of microbial contamination of catheter tips is significantly higher in individuals who present with an infection before IV therapy is begun than in non-infected patients. Take extra care to use aseptic technique with infected patients, both to prevent systemic infection via the IV catheter/ needle and to protect yourself and others with whom you come in contact.

6. The IV system

a. **Solution.** IV solutions especially those containing glucose, are excellent growth media for various microorganisms. Within 24 hours, Klebsiella and other gram-negative bacteria can multiply in glucose-containing IV solutions to levels that are likely to cause clinical sepsis. Reflux of blood into the tubing, or insufficient flushing of the line, may provide nutrients that allow additional species to thrive in the solution. Buffering of acidic dextrose solutions with bicarbonate likewise promotes the growth of additional organisms. The Centers for Disease Control make these recommendations for preventing infection:

- " . . . no intravenous bottle/bag should be left in place for more than 24 hrs"
- Bottles/bags should be closely inspected for the presence of cracks and punctures that are too small

to permit leakage but large enough to let bacteria in, and for turbidity and precipitation

- When there is suspicion that the fluid may be contaminated, the fluid should be cultured and the lot number noted
- Always check your expiration date on the IV solution prior to hanging

b. ***Administration set.*** Microorganisms capable of growing in IV solutions can live in IV tubing for days. Even when the infusion is continuous and rapid, bacteria are capable of ascending the tubing and contaminating the IV solution. Therefore, administration sets should be changed at least every 24 to 72 hours, and guarded against contamination at both the proximal and distal ends.

c. ***Dressings.*** Use of topical antibacterial preparations is likely to promote overgrowth of the yeast Candida and various resistant bacterial strains. Therefore, ointments are not recommended for use on an IV site. Agents such as povidone-iodine or Chlorhexidine Gluconate (Chloraprep®)—that kills not only bacteria but also fungi, protozoa, and yeasts are recommended for use for prepping and maintaining IV sites.

Note: The Chlorhexidine Gluconate prep is generally considered the best choice today because of less irritation to the skin and fewer allergic reactions. The Chlorhexidine Gluconate continues to act as an antibacterial agent for 48 hours under the IV dressing. Change a gauze dressing and apply new povidone-iodine solution or Chlorhexidine Gluconate every 48-72 hours. If a sterile transparent dressing is used, it may remain in place until the peripheral catheter/needle is changed (48 to 72 hours) as the site remains clean and dry. If the transparent dressing is used on a central line the dressing needs to be changed once a week and prn. If the dressing becomes wet, soiled, or otherwise contaminated, the area needs to be cleansed and new dressing applied.

d. Catheter/needle. Stainless-steel winged needles are thought by some to produce less infection than CON devices, but there is information refuting this claim. Winged needles tend to cause infiltration and have to be replaced more frequently. The Center for Disease Control recommends changing peripheral catheter/needles every 48-72 hours (this time may be longer if the catheter is made of an elastomeric hydrogel or other new material that increases the length of time the catheter may be left in place).

7. Blood

Septic shock resulting from transfusion of blood heavily contaminated with gram-negative bacteria is reported to carry a high mortality rate. The responsible organisms in these studies were mostly psychrophilic species, including Pseudomonas and coliform species. Fortunately, clinical infection from contaminated blood is quite rare. Four precautions help prevent infection:

- Use blood and blood products as soon as possible after they're taken from the refrigerator
- Discard the entire administration set after the transfusion
- Don't allow blood to hang for over four hours
- Avoid touch contamination of the blood and infusion system

B. MANAGEMENT OF SUSPECTED INFECTIONS

No matter how much care is taken, infections will occasionally develop as a result of IV therapy. Phlebitis at the puncture site is present in more than half the cases of infusion-associated septicemia, so phlebitis should immediately bring the IV system to mind when a patient develops a systemic infection (see Chapter 17). The IV system should also be suspected in the absence of noticeable phlebitis, especially if the catheter/needle has been in place for over 72 hours.

1. Determining whether septicemia is due to IV infusion

a. Obtaining culture specimens

- Culture IV sites and systems according to your facility's policies and procedures. Be careful not to contaminate the specimens during the collection process
- Carefully examine the insertion site; if it shows any sign of infection, take a culture sample
- Obtain blood samples from two separate venipuncture sites if the patient is febrile
- If possible, obtain blood culture specimens through the catheter to determine whether an infected thrombus is present
- Remove the entire infusion system, including the catheter/needle, and start a new infusion at another site (preferably the opposite limb)
- Send a sample of any fluid remaining in the system to the lab
- Send a culture of any pus or exudate from the site to the lab
- Cut the distal 1/3 to 1/2 of the catheter with sterile scissors, place it in the appropriate medium (according to the facility's policies and procedures), and send it to the lab

Note: The policy and procedure for performing blood cultures on a suspected catheter infection may vary from one facility to another. Check with your lab, physician or facility manual to determine the correct method for your facility.

b. Criteria for determining whether an infection is due to the IV infusion

- Culture positive for organisms at the insertion site
- Positive catheter-tip culture, with more than 15 colonies, if clinical evidence of infection is also present

- Purulent drainage at the insertion site
- Inflammation (redness, tenderness, swelling, warmth) at the insertion site without evidence of purulent drainage or cellulitis should **NOT** be regarded as infection unless a catheter-tip culture is positive

2. Treatment

The entire IV system (cannula, administration set, and fluid) is to be changed immediately if purulent thrombophlebitis, cellulitis, or IV-related bacteremia is strongly suspected or verified by blood cultures. All materials and the site are to be cultured appropriately. For phlebitis without signs of infection, the site should be changed immediately to the opposite limb if at all possible. Fortunately, infusion-associated bacteremias and fungemias often resolve spontaneously once the offending infusion system is removed. However, appropriate antibiotics should be given to the patient if clinical signs of infection or positive cultures persist.

3. Documentation

a. **Suspect products.** Record the nature and lot number of any suspect product. If evidence suggests contamination at the time of manufacture, local health authorities, the company from which the product was purchased and the Food and Drug Administration should be notified.

b. **Culture specimens.** Label each specimen with the following information:

- Patient's name and ID number
- Date and time
- Site from which the specimen was taken

c. **Charting.** Record the date, time and site of all culture specimens. When results come back from the lab, record them as well.

d. **IV therapy statistical records.** Record the patient's name ID number, date, time, site, and lab results for each culture specimen you take.

C. STANDARD PRECAUTIONS

a. Protective garments. It is vital that you wear whatever protective garment is necessary to protect you from contamination of any body fluids including, blood, secretions, excretions or contaminated waste products.

This may include:

Gloves: should be worn for

- touching blood and body fluids, mucous membranes, or non-intact skin
- handling items or surfaces soiled with blood or body fluids
- performing venipuncture and other invasive procedures
- Hands should be washed before donning gloves and after their removal
- Gloves should be changed after each patient contact

Masks and protective eyewear: should be worn for

- procedures that are likely to generate splashes or sprays of blood, body fluids, or other contaminated waste products

Gowns: should be worn during procedures that are likely to contaminate your clothing with blood, body fluids, or contaminated waste products

b. Needles and other sharp instruments.

Place all needles and sharp instruments in a puncture resistant container that can be closed and will not leak fluid. Do not:

- re-cap needles
- bend or break needles
- remove needles from the syringe or otherwise manipulate

- Needles and other sharp instruments should be placed in a red container or marked as biohazardous waste and disposed of according to your state's hazardous waste policy

c. Soiled dressings.

Dressings soiled with blood, secretions or excretions should be:

- placed in a plastic bag
- discarded according to your facility or state's hazardous waste policy
- If you pour a 1:10 bleach solution on the soiled dressings and close the bag it will aid in the decontamination process. Place the sealed bag into a second plastic bag, seal and discard.

d. Health care workers.

- Health care workers with exudative lesions or weeping dermatitis should refrain from direct patient care and from handling patient care equipment until the condition is resolved.
- Injury from a contaminated needle, or other sharp object, should be reported promptly to your supervisor or the employee health nurse for investigation, treatment if indicated and follow-up.
- If stuck with a contaminated needle stop and remove your gloves, make the wound bleed (you may wipe the wound with an alcohol wipe) then cleanse with soap and cool water.
- It is important for health care workers to stay current in their knowledge regarding guidelines for exposure to potentially contaminated substances, suggested precautionary measures, and treatments post exposure.

- Health care workers dealing with patients blood should receive the Hepatitis vaccine (Heptavax) for protection against Hepatitis B. This is a series of three injections and is generally covered by the employing agency. Once the series is completed the healthcare worker should have their titer checked on an annual basis to ensure that their titer remains at 10 or above. If their titer falls below 10 they should receive a booster injection.

NOTE: Some people fail to develop antibodies even after three or more injections. The series (3 injections) may be repeated a second time but if antibodies fail to develop, after the second series, the injections should be discontinued.

CHAPTER 22

Patients With Special Needs

Some patients require special needs because of the nature of their illness or the length of their required therapy.

A. LONG TERM IV THERAPY.

Patients requiring months or years of therapy will need special consideration regarding:

- **Venous access.** If therapy is anticipated to be lengthy, a stable, durable and reliable access route is required. It is best to address this issue at the onset of therapy rather than waiting to deplete all the patient's peripheral veins before considering a more permanent access. A long term central line is generally the best choice for long term infusion therapy.
- **Education.** If therapy is expected to continue for several weeks or longer, it will be important to identify someone to manage or assist with the care. This may be the patient or a designated caregiver that is willing and able to be taught.
- **Emotional response.** The psychological impact of long term IV therapy can be devastating to a patient and their family. Patients may become extremely controlling, demanding, depressed, withdrawn, etc. Allowing the patient to be as independent as possible, participate in their care and the

decisions relating to that care, to verbalize their feelings and even refuse continued treatment (being aware of the ramifications of that decision), are all important factors in helping to maintain their psychological well being. There may be times that additional professional counseling may be indicated and the nurse needs to be aware of the resources available for that patient.

B. IMMUNOSUPPRESSED PATIENTS

Patients may be immunosuppressed due to long term steroid therapy, chemotherapy, major trauma, a genetic disorder or HIV+. Regardless of the reason, these patients are at risk for many opportunistic infections (table 22-1). Education is the most important factor in helping immunosuppressed persons to maintain an optimal level of health. Education is also the primary factor in reducing the spread of infections. The following guidelines are suggested for use in educating patients, caregivers, and healthcare workers regarding healthy living practices.

1. General Hygiene

a. Hand washing is most important:

  - After use of toilet or contact with body fluids
  - Before preparing food or eating
  - Before administration of medication

b. Personal care

  - Body and hair kept clean—use a mild soap/shampoo
  - Maintain good oral hygiene—use a soft brush
  - Brush teeth after meals
  - Floss teeth if appropriate
  - Get regular check ups
  - Limit sweets
  - Check mouth daily for sores or white patches
  - Check body daily for skin irritations or sores
  - Keep nails short, clean and trimmed

c. Articles that should **NOT** be shared include:

-   thermometers
-   razors
-   toothbrushes/water picks
-   douche or enema equipment
-   any product that comes in contact with blood or body
    fluids

2. Bathrooms

Bathrooms may be shared if a few simple guidelines are followed.

a. Clean toilet, bathtub, shower, bathroom and floors with a freshly prepared solution of one part bleach to nine parts of water (1:10). If a toilet is splashed with urine or feces it must be wiped off then cleansed with the 1:10 bleach solution.
b. Sponges/rags used to clean floors or body fluid spills should not be used in eating areas and should be cleaned by soaking them for five (5) minutes in a bleach solution (1:10). When possible, use paper towels to clean up spills.

3. Kitchens

a. Eating utensils should be washed with hot water and soap
b. Clean the refrigerator and counter surfaces regularly with soap and hot water
c. Mop kitchen floor weekly or more often if necessary

Table 22-1. Infections frequently associated with immunosuppression

Organism	Manifestation	Treatment	Isolation/Precaution
Superficial Yeast Candida	Oral white patches Esophagitis May present in dis- seminated form in lungs	Nystatin orally (swish & swallow) Ketoconazole, Amphotericin	No isolation Employ meticulous hand washing after handling secretions
Systemic Yeast Cryptococcoses	Combination of site: Pneumonia, Meningitis, Lymphadenopathy, Endocarditis skin ulcers	Amphotericin Flucytosine	Secretion/excretions from in- fected sites should be handled with appropriate universal precautions
Fungal Coccidioidomycosis	Pulmonary lesions, skin lesions Disseminated — lungs, lymph nodes, CNS meningitis, GI organs	Amphotericin, Keto- conazole 6 mo. duration of therapy	Wound precautions with draining skin lesions
Blastomycosis	Pulmonary lesions — empyema, Cutaneous lesions, Disseminated CNS, bone, prostate	Amphotericin Hydroxystil- bamidine	Prevention of vector spread of respiratory secretions
Aspergillosis	Pulmonary infection sys- temic ENT, skin lesion, endocarditis, meningitis, kidneys	Amphotericin	No special isolation
Histoplasmosis	Disseminated to GI tract, oropharynx, hepatomegaly, splenomegaly, lymphadeno- pathy	Amphotericin Ketaconazole 6 mo. duration of therapy	No special isolation
Bacterial Mycobacterium avium Intracellulare	Disseminated — lung, liver, spleen	Dapsone Thiambutosine Clofazimine	No special isolation. Prevent secretion contact with resp. involvement.
Nocardiosis	Pulmonary lesions, brain abscess, skin lesions	Sulfonamides	No special isolation
Shigellosis	Diarrhea	Ampicillin Tetracycline, Pare- goric, Propantheline Lomotil, Imodium	Enteric Precautions — stool
Parasitic Pneumocystis carinii	Pneumonia — diffuse interstitial	TMZ-SMX, Penta- midine	With productive cough — respiratory — to prevent transmission to other im- munosuppressed residents
Toxoplasmosis	Nonspecific — asymptomatic to fulminating brain abscess hepatitis, encephalitis, myocarditis	Pyrimethamine, Sulfonamides	No special isolation
Viral Cytomegalovirus	Subclinical — pneumonia Retinitis, skin rash lymphadenopathy, hepa- tosplenomegaly	DHPG Foscarnate	Secretion/Excretion precautions
Herpes Virus	Disseminated mucocutaneous pneumonia, Encephalitis	Acyclovir Ara — A	Disseminated — Strict Local — Wound & skin, secretions from infected sites. Encephalitis — no isolation.

4. Food Preparation

People who are immunosuppressed can safely cook for others. They should follow the usual practice for safe food preparation. Since their immune system is altered, they are at greater risk for food poisoning and should be aware of safe food preparation and storage.

    a. Avoid unpasteurized milk
    b. Thoroughly wash fresh fruits and vegetables
    c. Cook chicken and all meats thoroughly
    d. Don't use cracked eggs
    e. Don't eat raw eggs
    f. Clean the outside of the eggs before breaking them open
    g. Cleanse the tops of cans before opening them up
    h. Keep foods refrigerated appropriately
    i. Don't lick fingers or taste from mixing spoon while cooking

5. Laundry and Linens

    a. Standard Precaution guidelines should be utilized when handling linens.
    b. Clothing or linen soiled with body fluids should be stored separately in a plastic bag. They should be washed separately in a washing machine using **HOT** water, detergent and bleach. Linens and other clothes not soiled by body fluids may be handled in the usual manner.
    c. Used towels and washcloths should not be shared. However, they can safely be used by others after they have been washed using the above laundering guidelines.

6. Trash Disposal

    a. Body wastes such as urine, feces and blood may be flushed down the toilet.
    b. Discard dressings, chux or any disposable material soiled with body secretions or blood into a plastic bag. Pour a 1:10 bleach solution onto the soiled material and seal. Place the sealed bag into a second plastic bag, seal and discard in the trash.

   c. Sharp items (needles, razor blades, etc,) should be placed in a puncture proof, leak proof container that can be securely sealed. Arrangements should be made with a hospital, health department or supply company for proper disposal of these items according to state/local law (incineration is the preferred method of disposal in most areas).

7. Smoking

   a. Smoking decreases the oxygen levels in the blood, predisposes the patient to heart attack, emphysema and cancer, depletes the body of vitamins and minerals and further suppresses the immune system

   b. Encourage the patient to stop or greatly reduce smoking

8. Exercise

Exercise should be tailored to meet the individuals ability with as much participation in ADL's as the patient can manage.

   a. Increases muscle tone and increases the circulation of healthy cells

   b. Mild to moderate exercise helps with sleep and assists in fighting depression, a known immunosuppressant

9. Immunizations

Immunizations should be kept current especially for Influenza (Flu), Pneumonia, Tetanus and Diphtheria. Regular checkups with the patients physician will help maintain and maximize the body's reserves.

10. Sleep

   a. 6-8 hours nightly

   b. A 1-2 hour nap may be needed during the day

   c. Too much sleep may be a sign of clinical problems or depression

11. Pets

Pets supply a great deal of love and affection but need to be cared for judiciously with great care.

    a. Pets that are exclusively indoor animals and isolated from other animals pose the least amount of risk
    b. Maintain the health of the animal by keeping up on immunizations and regular checkups at the veterinarians
    c. Immunosuppressed patients should not clean:

        - bird cages—a source of Psittacosis
        - cat litter boxes—a source of Toxoplasmosis
        - fish tanks—a source of mycobacterium

12. Intimacy

Physical touch is vital to psychological and physiological well being. Healthcare workers are in a "touching" profession and it is important to remember to reach out and touch our patients to let them know that we really care. Touching can be "healing". Don't wear gloves, etc. unless necessary. This only places another barrier between you and the patient.

    a. Safe sex should be practiced at all times
    b. Information, pamphlets and counseling should be made available as necessary regarding safe practices for intimacy
    c. Don't share sex "toys"

13. Positive Attitude

Depression is a known immunosuppressant and may be fought by encouraging the patient to stay as mentally and physically active as possible.

    a. Learn to be positive—set goals and aim for them
    b. Cherish each day—do something nice for yourself each day—learn to ask for what you need

c. Build your support systems—stay involved with family and friends; find new groups (peer groups, therapy groups or support groups)
d. Develop your sense of humor
e. Establish or further develop your spiritual life

14. Nutrition

a. Increase your intake of carbohydrates for energy. This will even your blood sugar levels and help prevent hypoglycemia.

   - carbohydrates: pasta, egg noodles, crackers, cereals, whole grain breads, potatoes

b. Vegetables: Increase your intake of vitamin B rich vegetables such as kale, broccoli, spinach and dark greens. Other vegetables such as carrots, beans, and cauliflower are also rich in vitamins and easily digested. Be cautious of tomatoes and peppers—they may be difficult to digest and cause sores in the mouth.
c. Fruits: Any fruit which can be tolerated easily is acceptable—citrus fruits, apples, pears, grapes, etc. Fruit juices are important for Vitamin C. If there are problems with digestion or diarrhea, citrus fruits may aggravate the system. Grapes or grape juice are a good supplement.
d. Proteins: Cheeses (low fat), milk (1%-2% or skim), poultry, fish, small amounts of red meat (beef), eggs (3-4 times per week), yogurt, tofu. Products low in fat are advised for easier digestion.
e. Supplements: Milk shakes or fruit shakes made with protein powder, low fat milk, honey, gatorade and/or fruit juice add additional nutrition.
f. Fluids: Maintain adequate hydration by drinking plenty of juices, Gatorade and water.
g. Sweeteners: Simple cane sugars, candy and sweets need to be eaten in limited amounts. Besides increasing chances of tooth decay, they can cause hypoglycemia and feed bacterial

infections like oral thrush. Use complex sugars like honey or molasses to sweeten foods.

h. Vitamins: A daily supplement of the following vitamins will help to increase the energy level, maintain healthy cells and prevent appetite loss.

- Multi-vitamin
- B-Complex
- C—(2000 mg minimum per day)

15. Preventing Cross Infections

Standard Precautions should be utilized for all patient contact.

a. Wear gloves when handling body fluids, linens or other objects contaminated with blood or body fluids: i.e. bathing, emptying a bedpan or commode, shaving with a safety razor, cleaning up body excretions, cleaning toilet fixtures, drawing blood or performing an invasive intravascular procedure (starting an IV, inserting a PICC line, accessing a PORT, etc.), giving mouth care, suctioning, changing wound dressings, etc.

b. Wash your hands before and after direct contact with any patient (after removal of gloves, if gloves are used).

c. Disposable gown or apron may be worn if necessary to protect your clothing from becoming soiled with blood or body fluids.

d. Mask should be worn:

- when in close contact (within 3 ft.) of a patient who has a productive cough
- if suctioning or performing a procedure that is likely to cause a spraying of body fluids or blood (goggles may also need to be worn for procedures likely to cause spraying)
- if the caregiver has a cold or flu

C. HOSPICE/CANCER/HIV+ PATIENTS

1. Hospice/cancer patients often have poor peripheral venous access. Chemotherapy, Radiation treatments, multiple infusions and blood tests have traumatized their veins to a point that their veins may be unavailable for peripheral access. The majority of hospice/cancer/HIV+ patients will need some type of central venous access device.

   a. PORTs are frequently utilized because of their ease of maintenance and no dressings required when they are not accessed.

   b. PICC lines are sometimes utilized because of their ease of insertion (they are frequently done at the patient's bedside), can remain in place for at least one year and do not require being "stuck with a needle" to access.

   c. Tunneled catheters are sometimes utilized because they can remain in place for many years, do not require being "stuck with a needle" to access, are easy for the patient or caregiver to use and maintenance is minimal.

2. Patient input when choosing the "type" of central venous access device to have placed will go a long way in patient satisfaction, compliance with therapy and care of the device. It gives the patient some control over what happens to them and they are more amenable to participating in their care.

CHAPTER 23

Pain Management

A. Pain is a major healthcare concern in the United States. More than 100 million Americans suffer from pain caused by various diseases and disorders, surgery and traumatic injuries. Pain is the most common reason individuals seek medical attention. The American Pain society (APS) reports that 50 million Americans have some level of disability caused by pain.

B. Although most pain can be relieved with proper management, it frequently is untreated, under treated or improperly treated. When untreated or ineffectively treated, pain prevents persons from leading a full and meaningful life, and leads to serious adverse health conditions, some which may even be fatal.

C. Joint Commission has implemented standards to help health care organizations provide effective pain management. **Pain *CAN* and *SHOULD* be controlled.**

D. As healthcare providers we hold to the principles that we will help our patients live their lives with quality and dignity. Since pain affects not only the quality of a patients life but also their dignity, we must address their pain issues if we are to put our words into action.

E. Today patients have the "Patient's Bill of Rights" which gives them:

1. The right to have their report of pain taken seriously and to be treated with dignity and respect.
2. The right to have their pain thoroughly assessed and promptly treated.
3. The right to receive a prompt response to unrelieved pain.
4. Their right to be informed and involved in all decisions regarding all aspects of their pain management.
5. The right to receive education regarding the management of their pain, treatment options and side effects.

F. Improper pain management has resulted in law suits with monetary awards to the aggrieved parties. Law suits focus on responsibility of health care providers to ensure that pain issues are addressed, the proper administration of pain medications and dosages are appropriate to control the patient's pain.

G. The benefits of pain control include:

1. Improvement in the quality of life
2. Improves mobility
3. Decreases depression
4. Improves socialization
5. Improves function and memory
6. Improves sleep

H. Pain in geriatric people (over 60 yrs. old) is frequently double that of younger people. Be aware of the sensitivity of geriatric patients to certain drugs (Beer's list).

I. Harmful effect of unrelieved pain include

1. Increased:

   a. ADH
   b. Hyperglycemia
   c. Heart rate
   d. Blood pressure
   e. Myocardial O_2 demand
   f. Anxiety

       g. Fear

       h. Stress

       i. Sleeplessness

       j. Hypoxia

  2. Decreased:

       a. Urinary output

       b. Gastric and bowel motility

       c. Mobility

       d. Activity, cognitive function

       e. Immune responses

J. Definitions

  1. American Pain Society: "Unpleasant sensory and emotional experience associated with actual or potential tissue damage, or described in terms of such damage."

  2. Bottom Line: Pain is subjective, complex and personal. Pain is whatever the patients says it is and occurs whenever the patient says it does.

K. Influencing Factors that affect a persons perception of their pain include:

  1. Medical history

  2. Past experiences

  3. Perceived level of pain

  4. Level of functioning prior to pain

  5. Disease process

  6. Age

  7. Culture

  8. Anxiety

  9. Coping skills

  10. Family role/expectations

L. You must know something about your patient to adequately assess their pain status and the treatment that would be appropriate. Be sure to include:

1. Review their drug & medical history (allergies/co-morbidities)
2. Possible side effects—constipation, gastric upset, sedation, nausea
3. Use of over the counter medications—especially Tylenol & NSAIDs, herbal and/or "home" remedies
4. Intensity of their pain (many scales are available to assist in this process)
5. Location/pattern of radiation to other areas
6. Quality/sensation (i.e. sharp, burning, stabbing, etc.)
7. Onset of pain and duration
8. Alleviating and aggravating factors
9. Current and past pain management modalities
10. Effect/impact on activities of daily living and sleep patterns
11. Their typical coping responses/methods
12. Their goal for pain relief

   a. It is important to know how much pain a patient expects to have or believes is "normal"
   b. When their goal is defined, it must be documented in the patient's record so all clinical staff will know if the management plan is on target or needs to be altered

M. Pain Assessment

1. The single most reliable indicator of pain is the patient's self report!
2. Failure to ask patients about their pain is the most common cause of unrelieved pain and unnecessary suffering. Do not wait for the patient to request pain medication. Regular and routine assessments should be done on all patients even if they are not complaining of pain.
3. Not everyone responds in the same manner to pain even though they may have the same type of background. Nurses usually report that "expressive" patients often come from Hispanic, Middle Eastern, and Mediterranean backgrounds, while "stoic" patients often come from Northern European and Asian backgrounds. Even though generalizations can be made we must be aware of the dangers of stereotyping.

4. It is important for healthcare providers to be aware of their own cultural and personal biases and how they may affect their response to patients in pain. Each patient must be treated as an individual. Honesty and respect are vital in obtaining an accurate assessment and establishing a trusting relationship with your patient.

5. ABC's of Pain Assessment

   a. Ask—about pain regularly and assess pain systematically
   b. Believe—the patient in their report of pain and what relieves it
   c. Choose—pain control options appropriate for the patient
   d. Deliver—interventions in a timely, logical, coordinated manner
   e. Evaluate their response to the treatment received and Enable the patient to control the course of their treatment as much as possible.

N. Pain Scales

A variety of pain scales are available and you will most likely need to use more than one type. Various scales may help you to identify the patients pain more accurately than others.

1. The verbal descriptor may be best used for patients who have difficulty with numbers. The words used can then be given a numeric value to identify the level of pain they are experiencing. Words such as No pain **(0)**; Mild **(1-2)**; Discomforting **(3-4)**; Distressing **(5-6)**; Intense **(7-8)**or Excruciating **(9-10).** The verbal descriptor scale is most often preferred by older adults.
2. Numeric scales **0-5** or **0-10** are frequently used effectively.
3. Wong-Baker Faces are frequently used with children or with adults with cognitive problems.
4. FLACC scale is frequently used with children and may be used for those who are unable to utilize the numeric or verbal scales to report their pain due to their level of mental development, cognition or emotional status. F=

Facial expression; L=Leg movement; A=Activity; C=Crying; C=Consolability.

5. Functional Scale (developed by Dr. Michael Gloth) is based on the patient's ability to perform various activities of daily living. **(1-2)** Tolerable (doesn't interfere with any activities); **(3-4)** Tolerable (Interferes with some activities but is bearable); **(5-6)** Intolerable (Still able to talk on phone, watch TV, read, sleep intermittently); **(7-8)** Intolerable (Unable to talk on the phone, watch TV, read, difficulty sleeping); **(9-10)** Intolerable (Unable to verbally communicate, talk on phone, watch TV, read or sleep) the worst pain you have ever experienced.

6. There are many pain scales available for use with cognitively impaired adults (i.e. CNVI, PAINAD, NOPPAIN, DS-DAT, Doloplus-2, PACSLAC, ECPA, PADE). You may need to try several different ones to see which fits your patients the best.

7. You will often need to be the "Pain Detective" to identify the true level of your patient's pain. Watch for non-verbal clues such as, guarding, moaning, grimacing, crying, decreased range of motion, decreased appetite, vital signs. They will often give you a fairly realistic reading of the level of pain your patient is experiencing. Some patients who have lived with chronic pain for a long time will not exhibit any of these signs and often endure rather high levels of pain before asking for medications.

8. Whenever evaluating a patient's pain always listen to what you patient is saying and objectively evaluate their vital signs and activities of daily living.

O. Classification of Pain—There are three classifications of pain.

1. **Acute Pain:** lasts less than 3-6 months and usually disappears when healing occurs of the cause is relieved. Pain medications need to be given more frequently with acute pain!! Some examples of acute pain are: surgery, traumatic injury; invasive procedures; childbirth.

2. **Chronic Non-malignant Pain:** Lasts longer than 3-6 months, or beyond the expected time for healing. It may be associated with a long term incurable or intractable

medical condition or disease. Some examples are: arthritis, fibromyalgia, neuropathy, reflex sympathetic dystrophy, crohn's disease, chronic pancreatitis, migraine headaches, back pain.

3. **Malignant Pain:** is pain associated with actual tumor or pain associated with the treatment of cancer, such as tissue damage caused by radiation therapy.

P. Key to Pain Control

1. 4 out of 5 patients have 2 or more types of pain.
2. Assess your patient thoroughly and accurately—what type of pain are you treating?

Q. Types of Pain

There are basically six categories of pain that most pain will fit into.

1. **Visceral/Soft Tissue Pain:** Primarily found in post-op patients, cancer patients, wound patients (especially stage III & IV), Necrotizing Fascitis.

   Patients will often describe this pain as:

   a. Constant—the pain is always there
   b. It hurts the same no matter is they are lying down, sitting or standing
   c. 100% Opioid responsive—may need an anti-inflammatory drug if tumor/disease process is causing inflammation.

2. **Bone Pain:** Frequently associated with decubitus, arthritis, fractures, metastasis, surgery on bones (i.e. hips, knees, spine). Bone Pain is semi-responsive to opioids. Generally a mild analgesic (i.e. Ultram) is often given along with an NSAID or Cox-2 inhibitor (i.e. Toradol or Celebrex—check contraindications for patient use). Precaution needs to be observed in giving an NSAID or Cox-2 to a patient with a

history of GI bleed, thrombocytopenia or renal dysfunction. Bone pain is often described as:

a. Intermittent pain
b. Worse with movement
c. Dull, steady ache
d. Throbbing

3. **Nerve Pain**

There are two types of nerve pain:

a. **Compressive nerve pain**—is semi-responsive to opioids. Generally a mild analgesic (i.e. Ultram) is often given along with an anti-convulsant (i.e. Neurontin or Tegretol ER) and/or an anti-depressant (i.e. Paxil, Elavil). Compressive nerve pain is often described as:

  ➢ Intermittent pain
  ➢ Stabbing
  ➢ Deep aching
  ➢ Gnawing
  ➢ Frequently triggered by movement
  ➢ **Often** radiates down the hip, leg or arm

b. **Neuropathic nerve pain**—is opioid resistant. Neuropathic nerve pain is frequently associated with diabetes and HIV+ but also includes fibromyalgia, phantom pain (post amputation), shingles, reflex sympathetic disorder and other causes of nerve damage. The best medication on the market at this time to treat this kind of pain is Lyrica (Pregabalin). Other medications (i.e. Paxil or Neurontin) have been used but are not always effective. Neuropathic nerve pain is often described as:

  ➢ Burning
  ➢ Feeling of pins & needles
  ➢ Stabbing sensation

> Stinging
> Deep ache

4. **Muscle Pain**—is opioid resistant. Is frequently associated with post-op surgery of the back, neck, knee, hip, etc. as well as other conditions (i.e. DJD, osteoporosis) and situations involving muscle injuries (i.e. sprains, MVA, etc.). Muscle pain is generally most responsive to muscle relaxants (i.e. Skelaxin, Flexeril, Soma), sometimes an NSAID and non-pharmaceutical interventions (i.e. massage, warm packs, etc.). Muscle pain is often described as:

> Sharp pain
> Cramping or grabbing feeling
> Intermittent pain
> Spasm
> Triggered by movement

5. **Colic Pain**—is opioid resistant. Often associated with irritable bowel syndrome, crohn's disease, colitis or nervous bowel. This type of pain frequently responds well to a anticholinergic or antispasmodic medication (these medications should **NOT** be given if ulcerative colitis is present). Sometimes an NSAID might help as well.

6. **Pleuritic Pain**—is semi-responsive to opioids. Since this is caused by an inflammation of the pleura surrounding the lungs an NSAID would be the first drug of choice along with a mild (i.e. Ultram) analgesic. Pleurisy often accompanies inflammatory lung disease, especially pneumonia. Pleuritic pain is often described as:

a. A grabbing sensation—especially with inspirations
b. Sharp—Stabbing
c. Intermittent pain

Pain Management Guide (see figure 23-1)—this guide can help you in identifying the type of pain the patient is having, how the patient will describe that pain to you, if the pain is responsive to opioids, semi-responsive to opioids or opioid resistant. Once you have identified the type of pain your patient is experiencing there are various drugs identified under each category to assist you determining what might be helpful to your patient. REMEMBER: 4 out of 5 of your patients may have more than one type of pain. Consequently they may require more than one type of medication.

Example: A patient with cancer is having a great deal of pain, he also has a history of arthritis and is diabetic with peripheral neuropathy. If you try to treat this patient with one type of medication you could render him unconscious and he would still feel pain. He will probably need 1. opioid (i.e. Morphine) 2. NSAID or Cox-2 for his arthritis pain (bone pain) and 3. Lyrica for his Neuropathic pain. *Most* of your patients will require *multi-modal therapy* to get them comfortable. This is preferred rather than giving them large doses of an opioid that makes them lethargic, sedated and doesn't control the pain. The synergistic effect of the use of various medications, designed to treat specific types of pain, is generally more effective than any one medication given alone.

Pain management. Pain may not be completely eliminated but the level should be tolerable for the patient. Analgesics should provide continuous pain relief and given in doses large enough to manage the pain without producing sedation. An intermittent medication should be ordered to allow for periods of breakthrough pain. A breakthrough dose of analgesic should only need to be given a maximum of 3-4 times in a 24 hr. period. When the breakthrough medication needs to be given more frequently, then the amount of continuous medication should be increased.

1. Pain is a very subjective and individual experience. Analgesics may be administered by several different routes including:

    ➢ by mouth (PO)
    ➢ intramuscular (IM)—should not be utilized for routine/ frequent administration of medications
    ➢ subcutaneously (SQ)
    ➢ rectally (PR)
    ➢ sublingual (SL)
    ➢ intravenous (IV)

➤ epidural
➤ intrathecal
➤ aerosol (inhalation/intranasal)
➤ transdermal (TD) The transdermal route (Duragesic patches) may not be as readily absorbed in extremely thin people because of a lack of adequate adipose tissue. The drug (Fentanyl) is absorbed through adipose tissue and should be placed over a fatty part of the body (i.e. upper arm, abdomen, etc.). Avoid placing it over bony areas. Without sufficient adipose tissue drug absorption may not be sufficient to control pain.

2. Factors that may influence the route selected:

➤ The patients history regarding the use of analgesics. A patient with mild pain who has a history of little or no previous use of analgesics will probably be easily controlled with small amounts of medication on an intermittent basis. A patient with a history of frequent use of narcotics (whether prescription or illegal) will have a fairly high tolerance for analgesics and will probably require higher doses of the analgesic, even for mild pain.

➤ The reason for the pain. If the patient has a condition where the pain is expected to diminish (e.g. surgery, trauma, etc.) the route selected may decrease in severity from one that is invasive in nature to one that is less severe in nature and frequency. If the disease process is one of progression, where pain is expected to increase, the route selected may increase from one of less invasiveness and intermittent in nature to one of more severity and continuous in nature.

➤ Individual, perceived level of pain. Pain thresholds are very subjective and individualized. Because of the nature of pain pre-established parameters are hard to establish and the nurse needs to monitor the patient closely to determine the therapeutic level of the analgesic.

3. The pain cycle. Patients typically experience a repetitive cycle of pain and sedation with the traditional intermittent methods of pain management, including intermittent PCA administration (see figure 23-2).

Figure 23-1

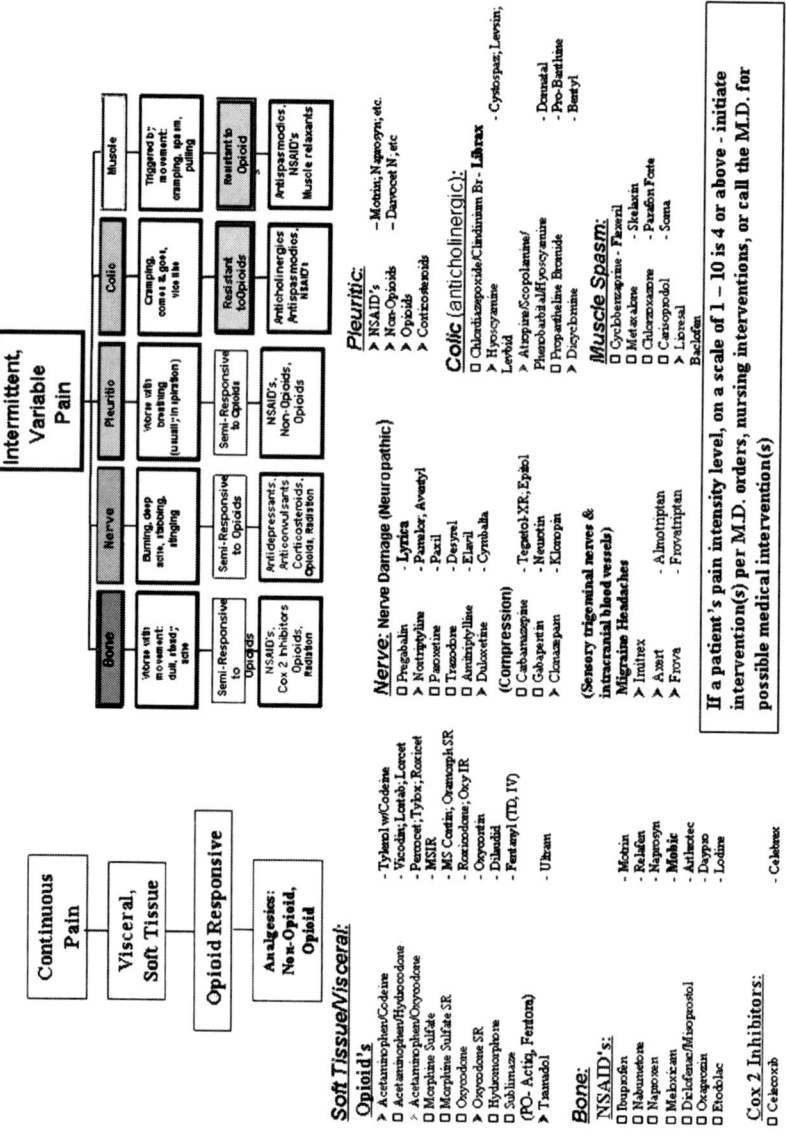

4. The continuous administration of an analgesic offers freedom from pain without the sedative effect (frequently with lower dosages). Even with a continuous administration of analgesic, additional bolus doses may be given for periods of "break through" pain. This method of pain management allows for optimal level of pain control. (Figure 23-3)

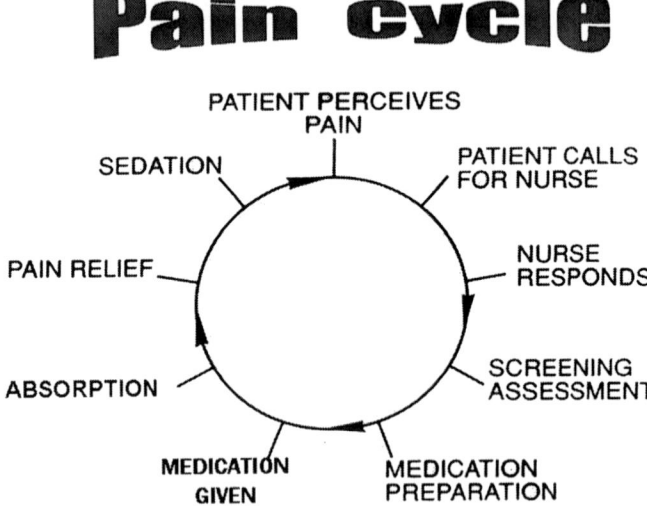

Patients typically experience a repetitive cycle of pain and sedation with traditional intermittent pain management practices.

Figure 23-2

Figure 23-3. Analgesic administration for optimal pain control

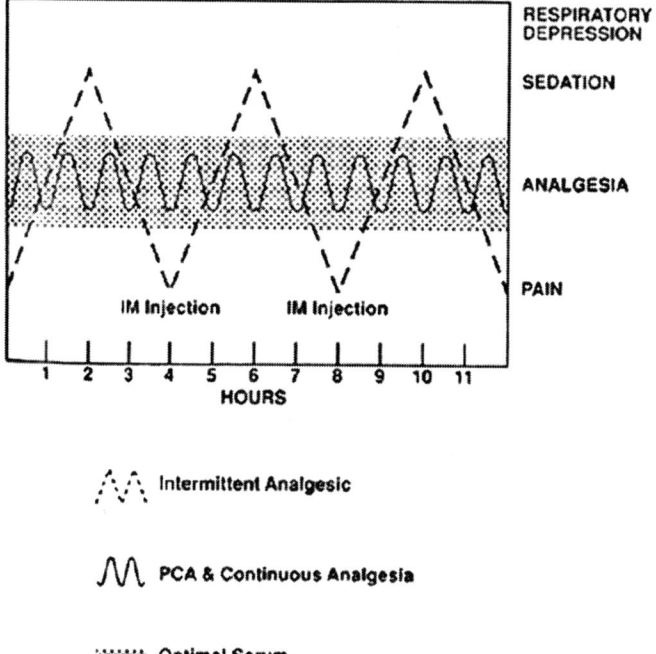

5. Studies have now proven that by giving an intermittent (PRN) dosing of pain medication you actually use **MORE** medication! Additionally intermittent dosing often results in:

   a. fluctuating effects of pain control & uncontrolled
   b. frequently under prescribed for the patient's needs
   c. puts the patient in a dependent role
   d. results in inconsistent responses to the patient by the nurse
   e. results in "lag" time between when the medication is called for and actually received
   f. patient differences not realized

6. If at first you don't succeed in relieving the patient's pain—try again, & again. Sometimes it takes several attempts to find the ***right drug*** that will work for the patient's pain and the ***right dosage***.

   REMEMBER: Your patient may have more than one type of pain—so may need more than one type of medication!!

7. Progressive Ladder for Pain Management (developed by the Oncology Nursing Society (ONS): Give the smallest dosage of the least potent drug you can give that will manage/control the patient's pain. When that drug/dosage is no longer effective, go to the next step (see figure 23-4). Increase the drug or amount sufficiently to control the pain or add another medication for additive or synergistic effect (see figure 23-1).

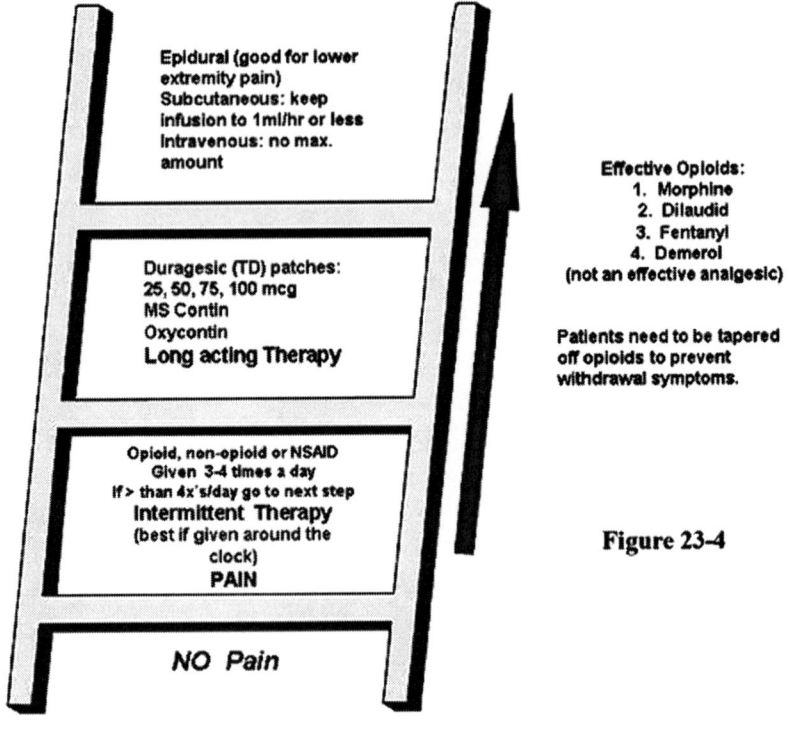

Epidural (good for lower extremity pain)
Subcutaneous: keep infusion to 1ml/hr or less
Intravenous: no max. amount

Duragesic (TD) patches: 25, 50, 75, 100 mcg
MS Contin
Oxycontin
Long acting Therapy

Opioid, non-opioid or NSAID
Given 3-4 times a day
If > than 4x's/day go to next step
Intermittent Therapy
(best if given around the clock)
PAIN

NO Pain

Effective Opioids:
1. Morphine
2. Dilaudid
3. Fentanyl
4. Demerol
(not an effective analgesic)

Patients need to be tapered off opioids to prevent withdrawal symptoms.

Figure 23-4

8. Candidates for long-acting opioid therapy:

   a. Patients with acute pain expected to persist over a period of time.
   b. Patients with chronic malignant pain.
   c. Patients with non-malignant pain expected to persist over a period of time (weeks/months/years).
   d. Use cautiously in patients with renal/hepatic insufficiency.
   e. If a short acting medication needs to be given more than q8hrs. or q6hrs. maximum, a long-acting medication needs to be given.
   f. Patients with a long-acting opioid will still need a short-acting analgesic to manage periods of break through pain.
   g. A long-acting opioid and a short-acting opioid may both be given at the same time. The short-acting provides pain relief until the long-acting is metabolized and can provide analgesia.

9. Subcutaneous Pain Management

   a. Subcutaneous injections:

      ➢ If given more frequent than Q 12 hrs., place a Subcutaneous needle
      ➢ If given more frequent than Q 2-3 hrs., evaluate the patient for a continuous infusion
      ➢ Works as effectively as IV
      ➢ May be administered continuously with or without a bolus dose
      ➢ ***Total dosage must be kept at a total volume of 1ml/hr.(includes continucus and bolus dosages)***

   b. Subcutaneous needles may be placed in the:

      ➢ Upper arms
      ➢ Anterior and lateral aspects of the thighs

> ➤ Abdomen
> ➤ Chest

  c. Subcutaneous site maintenance:

> ➤ Change site, needle and dressing once a week
> ➤ No flushes are required

10. Use of Patient Controlled Analgesic (PCA) pumps

  a. Should be considered for patients who are in constant severe pain

  b. May be programmed for continuous only, bolus only or continuous with a bolus

  c. Patients must have the mental capacity to recognize they are in pain and activate the bolus mechanism that interface with the bolus feature on the PCA pump

  d. The patient's use of the bolus dose should be monitored. If the patient needs to bolus more than 4-6 times in a 24 hr. period then the rate of the continuous infusion should be increased. This does not hold true for the immediate post-op patient. Their bolus is often set at q10 min. for a period of 24-72hrs. then decreased or discontinued.

  e. PCA bolus by Proxy should not be permitted—may cause a sentinel event

  f. PCA pumps may be utilized for IV, subcutaneous or epidural infusions

11. Special Patient Populations

  a. Renal Failure

> ➤ Avoid NSAIDs
> ➤ Decrease opioid dosage

  b. Hepatic Disease
> ➤ Decrease opioid dosage
> ➤ Avoid use of Acetaminophen
> ➤ Use NSAIDs with caution

c. Elderly patients

> ➤ Decrease use of NSAIDs
> ➤ Monitor opioid dosage closely in patients > 60 yrs. old

d. Chronic pain patients with opioid history

> ➤ Usually require increased opioid dosages
> ➤ NSAIDs may help ease the pain
> ➤ Adjuvant and non-pharmacological interventions may be helpful

12. Adjuvant Therapy

Adjuvant therapy should be considered whenever appropriate in **addition** to the analgesic to control the pain, anxiety or depression related to the disease process.

> ➤ Antispasmodics
> ➤ Anti-inflammatory drugs
> ➤ Anti-anxiety medications
> ➤ Anti-depressants

13. Always evaluate the effectiveness of the medication after it has been given. Generally evaluation can be done in 20-30 minutes if the medication was administered IV or subcutaneous and approximately 1 hour if administered PO.

Evaluate the level/intensity of the pain by frequently monitoring the appropriateness and effectiveness of the pain regime. Was the pain:

> ➤ Completely relieved (probably the right drug & dosage)
> ➤ Eased a little (probably the right drug but may need to change the dosage or add a synergistic drug)
> ➤ Not touched at all (probably the wrong drug). If it isn't working do something else!! and which pain?

14. **Over** medicating can be as bad as **under** medication. The right drug(s) and dosages should bring pain relief without sedating the patient.

15. Terminal Patients

> 68%-93% of terminal patients experience pain at the end of life.
> The principles of effective symptom control are always paramount. Diagnose the underlying cause of each symptom and tailor the treatment to individual circumstances and clinical context.
> Multimodal approaches to pain offers the potential benefit of additive and synergistic effects. Nine out of ten times the patient will need something for more than one type of pain.
> Pharmacologic and nonpharmacologic modalities need to be tailored to the individual likes, dislikes and effectiveness of the therapy.
> Normal pharmacokinetics and pharmacodynamics may be considerably altered by end-stage disease states.
> Inpatients with chronic liver disease or hepatic metastases, drugs may bypass hepatic metabolism altogether, increasing bioavailability.
> Renal clearance is almost always diminished during the dying process.
> To control pain in a "terminally" ill patient you may need to give extremely high doses of analgesic to get effective pain control.
> Patients with pancreatic cancer or metastasis, especially to the bone, will often have more pain than other types of cancer.
> Patients with bone metastasis should be on a steroid as well as their analgesic (opioid).
> There is **NO** upper limit for pain medications (patients often exceed 200mg of Morphine per hour). The patient should get whatever amount they need to be kept "comfortable". Monitor the

patient's vital signs and LOC to avoid respiratory depression.

16. Barriers to Effective Pain Control

a. **Addiction**—Patients should NOT experience a "high", euphoria, hallucinations, sedation or respiratory depression if the right drug and dosage are given. Addiction is characterized by behaviors that include one or more of the following:

  ➤ Impaired control over drug use
  ➤ Continued use of the drug despite harm
  ➤ Craving for a particular drug
  ➤ Multiple prescriptions from multiple doctors
  ➤ Doctor/hospital shopping

b. **Dependence**—A state of adaptation that is manifested by a withdrawal syndrome specific to the drug class.

  ➤ The syndrome can be produced by:

    o Abrupt cessation of the medication
    o Rapid dose reduction
    o Decreasing blood level of the drug
    o Administration of an antagonist (i.e. Narcan)

  ➤ Medication may be necessary to maintain pain control for the rest of the patient's life. This should not be an issue and the patient shouldn't be made to feel guilty (very common in malignant and chronic pain).
  ➤ Physical dependence does **NOT** equal addiction!! Evaluate the patient's use of the medication, their mental status, activities of daily living and is there are any s/s of an addiction process.
  ➤ Opioids used chronically for pain will cause dependence, but rarely addiction.

c. **Pseudoaddiction**—is misinterpretation of relief-seeking behavior as drug-seeking behavior.

  ➤ Develops as a consequence of inadequate pain management
  ➤ Behavior stops when adequate pain relief is provided

d. **Tolerance**—Once appropriate medications are identified and proper levels are reached the patient is generally stable. Increases are generally needed only when there is an exacerbation in the patients disease process or additional issues occur (i.e. Surgery).

e. **Lack of Knowledge**—Many healthcare practitioners are unaware of:

  ➤ Different medications needed for different types of pain
  ➤ Difference between chronic & acute pain
  ➤ Difference between addiction & dependence
  ➤ Benefits of multimodal therapies

17. Chronic Pain Patients

a. An accurate history is important to determine what the patient is using for baseline management of their pain. They often describe the duration of their pain in terms of months or years.

b. Generally require larger amounts of medication, above their baseline, for adequate pain control during periods of exacerbation or new issues.

c. Often do well with added adjuvant and non-pharmacological therapies.

  ➤ Diversional activities (massage, music, pets, aroma therapy, etc.) often decreases the intensity of the pain.

d. Don't always show alterations in BP and vital signs.

e. Are often very functional and may not appear to be in pain.

f.   Be alert for signs and symptoms of depression.

g.   Chronic pain issues:

> Peripheral vascular disease
> Post stroke syndrome
> Improper positioning
> Leg cramps
> Decubitus ulcers
> Contractures
> Headaches
> Amputation
> Reflex sympathetic disorder (RSD)
> Degenerative joint disease
> Arthritis
> Neuropathic pain
> Restless leg syndrome (RLS)
> Osteoporosis
> Myofascial pain
> Fibromyalgia
> Cancer
> Back pain

h.   Back Pain—a frequent chronic pain problem!!

> May be caused by:

   o   Disc disease/DJD
   o   Neuromuscular/ligament disorders
   o   Fractures (compression & traumatic)
   o   Facet disease
   o   Nerve inflammation

> Treatments:

   o   Pharmacological (i.e. Muscle relaxant + NSAID or Cox-2 or steroid + mild analgesic) may need something for nerve pain, if "radiation" down the arm or leg is present
   o   Non-pharmacological (Heat/Cold, exercises, massage, imagery, etc.)

o   Invasive treatments (Nerve blocks, Vertebroplasty, Sacroplasty, facet joint or sacroiliac joint injections)
o   Surgery

18. Patient/Caregiver Education

It is important for patients to understand why they are experiencing pain, that it is not something they have to endure and what pain management treatment options are available to them.

➤ Patients need to be actively involved in the development of their pain management plan of care.
➤ Patients and their families need to be aware that pain interferes with the healing process.
➤ Patients whose pain is not effectively managed have a slower recovery time and are less likely to actively participate in their rehabilitation activities.
➤ Patients should understand:

o   Signs and symptoms of reactions and side effects
o   Why we ask them to rate/describe their pain
o   The importance of effective pain management
o   Methods available to help ease their pain
o   The methods chosen and being used to manage their pain
o   To ask for their pain medication before the pain gets out of control
o   That if one drug or dosage isn't helping with their pain, other medications/dosages are available

19. Responsibilities in Pain Management

a.   Physician should order:

➤   the drug
➤   dosage
➤   route

> the rate—continuous vs. bolus or both
> adjuvant therapy—laxative, antiemetic, antianxiety, etc.

b. Nurse responsibilities

> Assess patient for signs/symptoms of pain
> Monitor for effectiveness of therapy regime
> Educate patient & family
> Consult M.D. for changes, as necessary
> Be an advocate for the patient's needs
> Document

c. Pharmacy responsibilities

> Fill medication as ordered
> Liaison with the facility, nurse & physician on pain issues

d. Equianalgesia chart (figure 23-5)

Equianalgesia

- *Provides equal analgesic when changing agents or routes of administration*
- **the nurse is the most likely one to convert the patient from parental to oral**
- **do not assume pain is less because patient is ready for different level of care**

Oral/Rectal Dose (mg)	Analgesic	Parenteral Dose (mg)
100	Codeine	60
-	Fentanyl	0.1
15	Hydrocodone	-
4	Hydromorphone (Dilaudid)	0.75
2	Levorphanol	1
150	Meperidine (Demerol)	50
10	Methadone	5
15	Morphine	5
10	Oxycodone	-

To switch routes of administration: USE HORIZONTAL AXIS
To switch between opioids: USE VERTICAL AXIS

Figure 23-5

20. Legal Issues

Documentation is the single most important factor in protecting you against litigation. You should document:

a. if the patient is having pain
b. level, location and type of pain
c. physician's orders
d. medication(s) given
e. effect of medication given (pain relief, sedation, etc.)
f. action taken—if treatment not effective
g. non-pharmacological interventions utilized
h. any communication with the MD/Pharmacy, etc.
i. patient/family education

CHAPTER 24

Home Infusion Therapy

A. Many intravenous therapy procedures may be done within the home care setting. These may include:

1. TPN & PPN (Nutritional Support)
2. Fluid & Electrolyte replacement
3. Antibiotics
4. Pain control (analgesics)
5. Chemotherapy
6. Blood/blood components
7. Dobutamine (cardiac perfusion)
8. IV push medications (eg. Lasix)
9. Cardiac drugs
10. Anticoagulants
11. Hormones

B. Illnesses which may benefit from Home Infusion therapy include:

1. Osteomylitis
2. Endocarditis
3. Wound infections
4. Systemic infections
5. Dehydration
6. Electrolyte imbalance
7. Cystic Fibrosis

8. Pneumonia
9. Crohn's disease
10. AIDS
11. Anorexia Nervosa
12. Failure to thrive
13. Pain
14. Carcinoma
15. Sporotrichosis
16. Congestive Heart Failure
17. Anemia
18. Septic arthritis
19. Prostatitis
20. Chronic congestive heart failure
21. Aspergillosis
22. Coagulation disorders
23. Diabetes
24. Ulcerative colitis
25. Hyperemesis Gravidarum of Pregnancy
26. Radiation Enteritis
27. Malnutrition
28. Hemophilia

C. Criteria for admission

Not all patients are candidates for home infusion therapy. Several factors need to be considered prior to accepting the patient for home care to produce a positive therapeutic outcome and a safe infusion environment. Factors that need to be considered include:

1. Geographic area—does the patient live within the designated geographic service area of your agency?
2. Reimbursement—how is the therapy, equipment and nursing care to be paid for? (eg. Medicare, Medical Assistance, private insurance, self-pay, indigent care, managed care)
3. Is the patient or a designated caregiver willing and capable of learning to:

   a. manage the infusion and equipment in the absence of the nurse?

    b.   understand the signs and symptoms of complications?

    c.   understand who and when to call for problems?

4. Participating Physician—a physician must be designated to assume responsibility for the care of the patient and provide orders necessary to effectuate that care. Also, the physician must be available as needed or provide adequate coverage in his/her absence.

5. Adequate planning

Many agencies have instituted the policy that the patient must have had the medication previously without any untoward reaction or receive the first dose of the medication in a controlled environment prior to accepting the patient for home therapy. In addition, the following considerations need to be addressed prior to initiating care:

    a.   Supplies—who will be responsible for the required components of care? (eg. medication and related equipment, pumps, pole, hospital bed and other Durable Medical Equipment required, nursing care, home health aide if needed, physical therapy, speech therapy or occupational therapy if necessary?)

    b.   Patient/caregiver education:

        -   teaching the use of equipment, drugs and possible side effects, complications, emergency procedures, universal precautions, disease process, etc.

        -   evaluation of the patient/caregiver comprehension and compliance with care

        -   documentation of the educational process and communication of the process to those involved with the patient's care (eg. M.D., PT, ST, OT, HHA, etc.)

    c.   Informed consent must be obtained prior to the initiation of care and should include:

        -   services to be rendered and their purpose

- possible complications and who should be contacted for problems
- who will assume the responsibility for care (the patient or a designated caregiver)?

d. Environmental factors to be considered include:

- is there access to a telephone?
- if medications are involved that need to be refrigerated, is refrigeration available and adequate?
- if a pump is to be utilized that requires electricity, is there electricity available and safe (grounded outlets)?
- household safety factors to review may include lighting, stairs, hallways, carpets, etc. depending on the therapy and equipment to be utilized in the delivery of that therapy.

e. Adequate venous access is vital to a successful course of intravenous therapy. If the patient is to receive his/her therapy via peripheral venous access, this should be evaluated prior to their release from the hospital or the initiation of their therapy. In the presence of poor peripheral venous access it may be advisable to address an alternate route that would be appropriate and meet the patients needs (eg. central line, subcutaneous infusion, PICC line, etc.)

D. Patient Care

Once a patient has been accepted for home infusion therapy, a continuous, dynamic process of planning, implementation and evaluation is set in motion to assure that the care provided meets the physician's orders, the patient's needs, regulatory standards and Insurance requirements. Components of this process include the following elements:

1. Plan of care—developed, with interdisciplinary input as appropriate, to address the needs of the patient and in conjunction with the patient/caregiver.

2. Patient/caregiver education and documentation of comprehension regarding:

    a.   purpose of therapy
    b.   patient/caregiver rights and responsibilities
    c.   medications, side effects, complications
    d.   equipment usage, complications, safety
    e.   disease process, universal precautions
    f.   emergency procedures

3. Monitoring of the patient's progress:

The intensity of the monitoring process depends on the nature of the illness, the therapy involved, the severity of the patient's condition and the patient/caregivers ability. The major components that need to be monitored on an ongoing basis will include:

    a.   improvement or deterioration of the patient's condition (including: physical, psycho-social assessments)
    b.   side effects or complications of medications/therapy
    c.   need for additional patient/caregiver education
    d.   need for ancillary services (O_2, DME, PT, ST, OT, HHA, etc.)

4. Communication and coordination of disciplines involved with the care:

If more than one discipline is involved with the patient's care it is imperative that communication between those entities be on-going and reflect the care provided/required and changes in care or patient condition. This may be in the form of:

    a.   written reports/orders
    b.   interdisciplinary conferences
    c.   verbal reports/orders

E. Nurse education/training.

The nurse providing infusion therapy within the home care setting should be trained and knowledgeable in the following areas:

1. General Principles of Infusion Therapy and Pain Management (as outlined in this book)
2. Regulatory requirements related to the practice of home care
3. Agency Policies and Procedures
4. Disease processes
5. Pharmacology—specifically those drugs that will be administered or that the patient is taking
6. Physical assessments—general systems review
7. Clinical dietetics
8. Infection control/Universal Precautions
9. Fluids and Electrolytes
10. Psycho-social aspects related to illness/home care

CHAPTER 25

Legal, religious, and psychological aspects of IV therapy

A. LAWS AND REGULATIONS

The legal ramifications of IV services provided to patients have significant implications for the personnel providing that care. Therefore, it is of paramount importance that all care providers be familiar with the laws and legal requirements surrounding the care they are providing regardless of the setting in which it is provided.

1. Personnel

   a. **State laws.** Different states have different laws concerning who may administer IV therapy. Certification authority for any nursing function rests with the state's board of nurses and the state's nurse practice act. Responsibility for this function may be delegated to other groups such as the state's nurses' association or may be handled by the state's board of consumer affairs. You should be familiar with these regulations and the limits they impose.

   b. **Institutional/Facility regulations.** Within each state, different institutions/facilities may have different policies regarding who may administer IV therapy. Increasingly, such policies are detailed in written IV Policy and Procedure manuals. In addition to specifying who can administer IV infusions, there may be policies governing procedures such as blood transfusion, placement of central lines, and injections of IV medications. It is essential that the facility develop its standards, policies and procedures in accordance with Federal and State regulations, established guidelines within the field and evidence based practice.

2. IV manual

Your institution's IV manual probably contains detailed descriptions of the following:

- Personnel—who is allowed to perform what procedures
- The equipment to be used in each type of procedure
- Verifying patient's identities
- Obtaining of consents
- Hand washing/Universal Precaution requirements
- Procedures for prepping/dressing IV sites
- How to perform each IV procedure
- Disposal of used IV equipment
- Maintenance of IV lines/sites
- How to use specialized equipment, and who is permitted to do so
- Infusion times for various medications
- Special instructions for various areas such as the ICU/CCU, emergency department, home care or out-patient departments. Note: Other resource Manuals printed by various companies are often utilized by facilities as their resource for certain Policies & Procedures. This often saves them a great deal of time from having to develop/write their own. If a facility is using a resource book for its P&P's the nurse should have access to the book for purposes of reference/verification.

3. Education of Health care personnel.

Additional training/education is frequently required for new or advanced therapies, equipment or technology. Health care providers should make **every effort to remain current within their field**

of practice and to practice within the scope of their license and training.

4. Documentation

Only complete and accurate records will serve the medicolegal needs of your patients, the hospital, physicians, hospital staff, and you. Your greatest protection against litigation is your documentation.

> *a.* ***What to chart.*** No matter how routine or insignificant something may seem to be, you should write it in the patient's permanent record. Legally speaking, if something is not charted, it is considered not done. Documentation should include:
>
> - Plan of care and medications—with changes as necessary to maintain a current profile
> - Never stick a patient without documenting it and the number of attempts, regardless of your success
> - notes of care provided for the patient with appropriate M.D. orders and changes as necessary
> - Education of the patient/caregiver, their comprehension and compliance
> - Patient response to treatment
> - Communication with family and all care givers
> - Any untoward incidents or complications
>
> *b.* ***Erasures.*** A patient's record is a legal document. Write everything in ink or input into the documentation computer. Never use correction fluid or erase anything you write. If you make an error, ink a line through it write "error" above it, include the date and your initials, and then insert the correct information.
>
> *c.* ***Objectivity.*** Keep your charting as objective as possible. Use quotation marks for direct quotes and statements of opinion by others. Attribute all quotations. Use word like "appeared" and "alleged" when writing about things that you did not witness or haven't been proven (verified).

5. Legal liability

   a. **Responsibility.** You are responsible for your own acts and can be sued for negligence if you fail to act in accordance with the standards set by your institution and the state board of nurses. Standards of practice, as stated by professional organizations and other health-care providers, are frequently utilized in determining the standard of care in any given area for a particular service or specialty.

   b. **Errors of omission.** Errors of omission can be just as detrimental as errors of commission. Failure to act prudently, in accordance with your knowledge and training, could result in a legal judgment against you.

   c. **Good Samaritan laws.** You cannot be found liable if you aid a person in distress unless you:

   - Exceed the limits of your training
   - Commit an act of gross negligence
   - Charge for your services

   In giving emergency care, you'll decrease your chances of being sued if you take the following steps:

   - Keep up your certification, skills, and knowledge
   - Defer to the person on the scene who has the highest level of training
   - Follow up with the patient if you were the person in charge during the emergency

   d. **Patients' rights.** Patients have certain rights that must be considered and protected. Many states have incorporated patients' rights into some form of legislative or administrative code. These "rights" frequently include the following, but check with your state authorities to determine your exact obligations concerning patients' rights in your area.

   - Considerate and respectful care provided without regard to gender, cultural, economic, sexual orientation, educational, or religious background

- Knowledge of the patient's primary-care physician and information from his physician about his illness, proposed course of treatment, and prognosis
- Receipt of information regarding any proposed treatment and/or specific procedures, and active participation in the decisions regarding the patient's own care—including the right to refuse any treatment or procedure
- confidential treatment and privacy concerning all communications and records regarding the patient's medical care
- Ability to leave the hospital "against medical advice" (AMA), unless being detained on a legal restraint
- Knowledge concerning all hospital/agency rules and regulations that apply to the patient's care/conduct
- Reasonable responses to reasonable questions regarding the patient's care and requests for service
- Being advised if the hospital/agency or physician proposes to engage in or perform human experimentation affecting the patient's care or treatment (the patient has the right to refuse to participate in such research projects)
- Being informed of the patient's continuing health-care requirements following his/her discharge from your service
- Examination of the patient's bill and receipt of an explanation of the costs regardless of source of payment

B. RELIGIOUS BELIEFS

1. Respect

Patients have the right to receive respect for all their religious beliefs. Before initiating IV therapy or pain management medications/ procedures, explain to the patient what you're going to do, and why. If the patient has concerns based on religious persuasion, a simple explanation may clear up misunderstandings and reassure him/her. If, after a thorough explanation, the patient refuses to accept treatment or undergo a procedure, that refusal must be respected unless it's overruled by a court decision. Notify the patient's physician of the refusal and document your actions and the physicians response in the patient's record.

2. Objectivity

Never let your own beliefs affect your attitude toward a patient.

3. Religious beliefs concerning IV therapy and medical treatment:

a. Jehovah's Witnesses. Members of this religion do not believe in blood transfusion or the administration of any blood product, including plasma and albumin. These individuals will usually cooperate if assured that an IV doesn't contain any blood product. In a test cast in 1980, a Jehovah's Witness accepted infusion of an artificial product capable of transporting oxygen.

b. Christian Scientists. Christian Scientists attain various levels of religious experience. Those who feel they've reached a high level of "science awareness" may refuse to accept any form of medical assistance.

c. Other beliefs. Some people believe that admission of pain or debility is a human weakness and reflects lack of religious faith. Others believe that by enduring pain they can transcend their bodies and attain a higher state of being in the afterlife. Still others believe that pain and suffering are God's punishment for their sins. Individuals with beliefs of these sorts may refuse IV therapy, pain medications and other forms of medical treatment.

C. PSYCHOLOGY IN IV THERAPY

Trauma, disease, and medical equipment are everyday encounters for you, but they may be new and very frightening experiences for patients. In addition to the pain, discomfort, and debility caused by the patient's physical condition, the experience of being in a hospital or the feeling of losing control of one's life and of one's individuality may produce a great deal of psychological stress.

1. Emotional crisis

a. Types of crisis. A crisis is an emotionally significant event or radical change in one's life. There are two types of medical crisis:

- **Expected**—when the patient has been ill for some time and their condition has slowly been deteriorating
- **Unexpected**—when sudden trauma or illness strikes

b. Stages of a crisis

- **Impact**—usually seen by emergency personnel—strikes at the moment of crisis
- **Recoil**—usually seen by healthcare personnel after the initial stage of impact has become a reality
- **Post-trauma**—seen by healthcare personnel and by the patient's family after discharge

c. Resolution. An emotional crisis is usually resolved by one of the following approaches:

- Problem solving
- Redefinition
- Adoption of a defense mechanism: denial, rationalization, etc.

2. Persons involved in a crisis

Three categories of people are generally involved in a crisis:

- The person experiencing the crisis—the patient
- Significant others—family, loved ones, close friends
- Onlookers—emergency and healthcare personnel, casual friends, interested bystanders, thrill seekers

Your task is to meet the immediate, life-threatening needs of the patient and to provide calm, objective support for the patient and his/her significant others.

3. Reactions to crisis and pain

a. Individual coping mechanisms. Everyone learns various ways of coping with situations that are frightening, painful, unexpected, embarrassing, suspenseful, or otherwise uncomfortable. To a certain extent, ethnic, cultural, religious, and socioeconomic factors determine how individuals cope with crisis and pain. A few commonly utilized mechanisms for coping are:

- **Conversion:** Conversion operates wholly on an unconscious level and allows the patient to convert strong emotional conflicts into physical symptoms (hysterical paralysis, headaches, GI symptoms, etc.).
- **Denial:** A patient may simply reject the fact of his illness or crisis. This is seen fairly often on medical and surgical units, and could have serious consequences for the patient with a major health problem. Patients coping through denial often retreat into themselves, become quite withdrawn and often refuse medications and treatments.
- **Displacement:** The transference of emotion from one object, situation, or idea to another (e.g., being angry with "God" or "fate" because of particular crisis or disease, and yelling at and blaming the nurse or doctor for the problem).
- **Identification or introjection:** Acceptance of a person, idea or object, feeling as though it is a part of one's self.
- **Projection:** The act of attributing unacceptable faults, failures, thoughts, or activities within the person to others in order to protect ones "self." This is frequently exhibited in angry shouting, inappropriate accusations, and demanding behavior.

- **Rationalization:** A method of self-deception, it is simply finding a logical reason for the things one wants to do.
- **Reaction formation:** The process of overcompensating for a negative feeling or activity by overdeveloping the opposite behavior. Someone who is overly sweet and polite may be attempting to disguise an underlying hostility. Inappropriate humor or joking may be covering up underlying fear.
- **Regression:** A common form of coping frequently found in hospitals. Regression occurs when the patient reverts to previous patterns of behavior that were successful in earlier stages of development (temper tantrums, crying, attachment, etc.).
- **Repression:** A patient actively forces unpleasant or unacceptable facts or experiences into his/her unconscious mind. The facts and/or experiences really can't be remembered. Repression operates wholly on an unconscious level.
- **Sublimation:** The act of substituting an acceptable activity (e.g., chewing gum) for an unacceptable one (e.g., smoking).
- **Symbolization:** A mental mechanism of the subconscious in which one idea or object stands for another.

b. **Physiological effects.** The physiological changes produced by the patient's physical condition may be made better or worse by his/her emotional reaction to the stress of crisis and/or pain—for example, loss of appetite due to depression or venospasms due to fear of being stuck with a needle.

c. **Reactivation of unresolved emotions.** The stress of crisis and pain may bring to the surface unresolved fears, anxieties, or problems that the patient had previously managed to suppress. This response is especially likely to happen when the patient subconsciously perceives a similarity between a stressful incident in the past and the present crisis. Bear this in mind when a patient appears disoriented or displays inappropriate behavior; he/she may be reliving a traumatic episode from the past.

4. Perception of pain

The degree and quality of pain perceived by the patient is as variable as other sensory perceptions. Even more variable may be the degree and manner of patients' expression of pain.

5. Your treatment of the patient

a. ***Acceptance.*** Accept the patient and family as they are. Acceptance doesn't mean approval. Acceptance of the present situation also doesn't mean that you won't accept changes in emotional outlook and behavior when they occur.

b. ***Listening.*** Let the patient and significant others ventilate their thoughts and feelings, both overt and covert. Sometimes covert signals (inflections in the voice, gestures, body language, etc.) are more significant in uncovering the "truth" about thoughts and feelings than is the overtly spoken word. ***ALL behavior has meaning.*** It is important that we develop a sensitivity to others' thoughts and feelings (both covert and overt) in order to understand the meaning behind the behavior. If we are to be effective in helping others to cope with their present problems and situations, and to proceed beyond the crisis of the moment to a healthy resolution and acceptable behavior, we must be "tuned in" to them by watching, listening, evaluating, and understanding the true essence of their thoughts and feelings.

c. ***Objectivity.*** Keep your own feelings out of your relationships with patients. Watch not only what you say but also how you say it. Be friendly and courteous; don't be afraid to be human and show that you care.

   - Empathy is an integral part of caring. If you can't be objective in dealing with a particular patient, ask someone else to care for him/her if at all possible. If you don't, chances are that you will probably reveal to that patient, in a covert manner, your dislike for him/her. This may have a negative effect not only on the patient but on you and other members of the health-care team.

Definition of empathy: an objective awareness and insight into the feelings, emotions, and behavior of others, and their meaning and significance.

d. **Confidentiality.** You should never discuss a patient's condition with others without the patient's consent. Never pass judgment or imply any deprecation of other health-care personnel or previous treatment in front of a patient or family members. Be careful not to discuss a patient's problems or condition in public places where family members, friends, or visitors may hear you (e.g., elevators, cafeteria, lobby, social gatherings). A patient's medical care, history and record are private and confidential. It is imperative that all health-care providers adhere to the confidentiality of their patient's care.

The passage of the Health Insurance Portability and Accountability Act (HIPPA) emphasizes the importance of patient healthcare privacy by making it a legal imperative.

6. Minimizing anxiety

You can do a great deal to minimize a patients' fears just by following these simple steps.

a. **Explain.** Always tell the patient who you are and what you're going to do. Encourage questions; the patient may have misconceptions about IV therapy, methods for relieving pain and other medical/surgical procedures learned from television or other sources.
b. Be friendly, courteous, and supportive.
c. Prepare equipment out of sight. Try to do as much preliminary preparation as possible out of the patient's sight and hearing. This usually helps minimize anxiety concerning the appearance and use of "strange looking" equipment.
d. Respect the patient's decision regarding his/her care.

D. SELF CARE AND UNDERSTANDING

Because of the intense nature of providing high-tech (infusion therapy), pain management and other medical services to patients who are frequently seriously ill and in need of a considerable amount of care, it is important for healthcare personnel to learn how to take care of themselves. The "Burn Out" rate among healthcare providers is extremely high and threatens to eliminate from the field many who honestly care and are trained and experienced in advanced therapies and treatments. We are excellent caregivers for others but frequently ignore our own needs before we are physically and emotionally exhausted. If we are to remain in the field for an extended period of time, where we are greatly needed to help our patients and help train other caregivers, we will need to learn the "art" of caring for our own needs.

1. **Awareness.** The first thing we need to do is to be aware of where we are. There are two key dimensions to pending burn out.

    a. **Demoralization**—feeling bad: we feel helpless, challenges become burdens and the process seems futile.

    b. **Diminished caring**—feelings of "they"ness versus "we"ness: we tend to detach ourselves from the caring process.

Some signs and symptoms that may indicate impending "Burn Out":

- fatigue
- sleep disturbances
- changes in appetite
- gastro-intestinal problems
- muscular tension
- headaches
- depression
- frustration
- anger and resentment

- obsessions
- feeling overwhelmed
- feeling inadequate
- decreased humor (cynicism)
- decreased caring
- feeling guilty
- increased alcohol or drug use
- avoiding responsibilities
- interpersonal conflict
- decreased productivity
- withdrawal (isolation)
- chronic lateness
- criticism of peers
- overreaction
- irritability
- resentment
- disorganization
- reluctance to go to work

2. Steps to healing and healthy living.

In order to begin the process of healing ourselves and learning to live in a healthy manner, we need to begin an active program to deal with our own needs and frustrations. Ten steps we can take to help with this process include:

a. Develop a strong support system: individual(s) you can share your feelings with in complete openness and honesty, that will accept you as you are without judging, rejecting, or trying to fix you.
b. Practice the art of the possible:

- do what we can to change the things we can change
- accept the things we cannot change

c. Find a healthy "escape hatch": a mechanism to release the internal tension and frustration (e.g., sports, jogging, music, arts, crafts, etc.)

d. Laughter. Learn to play and laugh. Science has proven that laughter is very healing to the physical as well as the psychological aspects of humankind. By cultivating our ability to laugh, it is possible to bring balance and perspective to life that will recharge and energize all our activities.

e. Rest. Burning the candle at both ends will burn you out fast! Take time to rest, meditate, and smell the flowers. Being cognizant of the beauty around you will go a long way in "recharging" your battery. Rest your body, mind and spirit.

f. Allow yourself to feel good about who you are and the profession you have chosen. If you are experiencing "burn out", it means you must have been on fire, at one time! You really care! That is a positive characteristic that deserves to be recognized and applauded.

g. Perform at least one act of kindness every day for YOURSELF! A fifteen minute walk in the sunshine, listening to a musical selection, read a book, take a warm bubble bath, purchase flowers for yourself, play a game with a friend, etc. are all good examples of acts of self-kindness that can help us to keep our balance.

h. Cultivate an active spiritual life.

i. Develop an attitude of appreciation for the things we have instead of focusing of the things we don't have. Accept, and internalize the praise offered by others as a positive affirmation of your inner caring and worth.

j. Learn to reach out to others for help and be willing to accept that help for yourself when it is needed.

So often we are more than willing to give and do for others but find it difficult to accept help from others for ourselves when we need it. By practicing these steps we can begin to get a healthy perspective on a program of "caring" for ourselves (the caregiver). Caring for ourselves will not only result in a healthier and happier self image but will enable us to continue providing loving care to our patients for many years to come.

BIBLIOGRAPHY

Anderson AO, Yarley JH. 1972. Demonstration of Candida in blood smears. *N Engl J Med* 286:108.

Ansel, HC, Gifandet MP. 1971. Change in pH of infusion solutions upon mixing with blood. *JAMA* 218:1052.

Banks DC, Tates DB, Cawdrey HM, et al. 1970. Infection from intravenous catheters. *Lancet* 1:443.

Bernard RW, Stahl WM, Chase RM. 1971. Subclavian vein catheterizations: A prospective study. II. Infectious complications. *Ann Surg* 173: 191.

Boeckman CR, Krill CE Jr. 1970. Bacterial and fungal infections complicating parenteral alimentation. *J Pediatr Surg* 5:117.

Bolasny BL, Martin CE, Conkle DM. 1971. Careful technique with plastic intravenous catheters. *Surg Gynecol Obstet* 131:1030.

Bolasny BL, Shepard OH, Scott HW, et al. 1970. The hazards intravenous polyethylene catheters in surgical patients. *Surg Gynecol Obstet* 130:342.

Braude AI. 1958. Transfusion reactions from contaminated blood, their recognition and treatment. *N Engl J Med* 258:1289.

Braude AI, Carey FJ, Siemienski 3. 1955. Studies of bacterial transfusion reactions from refrigerated blood: Properties of cold-growing bacteria. *J Clin Invest* 34:311.

Braude AI, Sanford JP, Bartlett JE, et al. 1952. Effects and clinical significance of bacterial contaminants in transfused blood. *J Lab Clin, Med* 39:902.

Brennan MF, O'Connell RC, Rosol JA, et al. 1971. The growth of Candida albicans in nutritive solutions given parenterally. *Arch Surg* 103:705.

Brereton RB. 1969. Incidence of complications from indwelling venous catheters. *Del Med J* 41:1.

Center for Disease Control. 1971. Nosocomial bacteremias associated with intravenous fluid therapy—USA, *Morbid Mortal Weekly Rep* 20.

Chaffee EE, Greisheimer EM. 1974. *Basic Physiology and Anatomy, 3rd ed.* Philadelphia: Lippincott.

Cheney FW, Lincol JR. 1964. Phlebitis from plastic of intravenous catheters. *Anesthesiology* 25:650.

Collins RN, Braun PA, Zinner SH, et al. 1968. Risk of local and systemic infections with polyethylene intravenous catheters. *N Engl J Med* 279:340.

Colvin MP, Blogg CE, Savage TM, et al. 1972. A safe long term infusion technique? *Lancet* 2:317.

Corso JA, Agostinelli R, Brandriss MW. 1969. Maintenance of venous polyethylene catheters to reduce risk of infection. *JAMA* 210: 2075.

Crenshaw CA, Kelly L, Turner RJ, et al. 1972. Bacteriologic nature and prevention of contamination to intravenous catheters. *Am J Surg* 123:264.

Duma RJ, Warner JB, Dalton HP. 1971. Septicemia from intravenous infusions. *N Engl J Med* 284:257.

Felts SK, Schaffner W, Melly MA, et al. 1972. Sepsis caused by contaminated intravenous fluids: Epidemiologic, clinical and laboratory investigation of an outbreak in one hospital. *Ann Intern Med* 77: 881.

Fisher EJ, Maki DG, Eisses J, et al. 1971. Epidemic septicemias due to intrinsically contaminated infusion products. *Abstr 11ᵗʰ Intersci Conf Antimicrob Agents Chemother (Atlantic City)*, p 20, October 20.

Freeman R, King B. 1972. Infective complications of indwelling intravenous catheters and the monitoring of infections by the nitroblue-tetrazolium test. *Lancet* 1:992.

Fuchs PC. 1971. Indwelling intravenous polyethylene catheters. Factors influencing the risk of microbial colonization and sepsis. *JAMA* 216:1447.

Fundamentals of Body Water and Electrolytes. 1974. Deerfield, Ill: Baxter Laboratories, Division of Travenol Laboratories Inc.

Gesco International Co., San Antonio, Texas

Glover JL, O'Byrne SA, Jolly I. 1971. Infusion catheter sepsis: An increasing threat. *Ann Surg* 173:148.

Goldfarb IW, Yates AP. 1980. *Total Parenteral Nutrition Concepts and Methods.* Pittsburgh: Synapse Publications.

Goldmann DA. 1972. Prevention of infection in hyperalimentation therapy. 9ᵗʰ *Int Cong Nutr (Mexico City)*, Sept 3.

Gray. 1974. *Anatomy, Descriptive and Surgical.* Philadelphia: Running Press.

Habibi B, Salmon C. 1972. Septic shock from bacterial contamination of transfused blood. *Lancet* 2:830.

Horshal VL. 1972. Intravenous catheters and infection. *Surg Clin North Am* 52:1407.

Insights Into Parenteral Nutrition. 1977. Deerfield, Ill: Travenol Laboratories, Inc.

James JD. 1959. Bacterial contamination of reserved blood. *Vox Sang* 4: 177.

Krauss RN, Albert RF, Kannan MM. 1970. Contamination of catheters in the infant. *J Pediatr* 77:965.

Levy RS, Goldstein J, Pressman RS. 1970. Value of a topical antibiotic ointment in reducing bacterial colonization of percutaneous venous catheters. *J Albert Einstein Med Cent* 18:67.

Lowenbraun S, Young V, Kenton D, et al. 1970. Infection from intravenous "scalp vein" needles in a susceptible population *JAMA* 212:451.

Lower Incidence of Peripheral Catheter Complications by Use of Elastomeric Hydrogel Catheters in Home Intravenous Therapy Patients. Journal of Intravenous Nursing, Vol. 14, No. 4 July/Aug. '91. J.B. Lippincott Co.

Maintenance Peripheral Nutrition. 1976. Deerfield, Ill: Travenol Laboratories, Inc.

Maki DG, Rhame FS, Goldmann DA, et al. 1973. The infection hazard posed by contaminated intravenous infusion fluid. In *Clinical and Laboratory Aspects of Bacteremias: A Symposium* (Sonnenwirth AC, ed). Springfield, Ill: Thomas.

Maki DG, Rhame FS, Mackel DC, et al. 1971. Nosocomial sepicemias subsequent to contaminated intravenous fluid. *Proc Annu Meet Am Soc Microbiol (Minnesota)*, May 5.

Managing I.V. Therapy. Horshani, Pa. 1982. Intermed Communications (Nursing Photobook Service).

Matheney RV, Topalis M. 1970. *Psychiatric Nursing, 5ᵗʰ ed.* St. Louis: Mosby.

Mays ET. 1972. A microbiological investigation of percutaneous central venous catheters. *South Med J* 65:830.

Meng HC, Wilmore DW, 1976. *Fat Emulsions in Parenteral Nutrition.* Chicago: American Medical Association.

Menlo Care, Inc. Palo Alto, California

Michaels L, Ruebner B. 1953. Growth of bacteria in intravenous infusion fluids. *Lancet* 1:772.

Moore FD, Brennan MF. 1972. Intravenous feeding. *N Engl J Med* 287:862.

Morgensen JV, Frederiksen W, Jensen JK. 1972. Subclavian vein catheterization and infection: A bacteriologic study of 130 catheter insertions. *Scand J Infect Dis* 4:31.

Morton HD. 1968. Alcohols. In *Disinfection, Sterilization, and Preservation* (Lawrence CA, Black SS, eds), p. 237. Philadephia: Lea & Febiger.

Norden CW. 1969. Application of antibiotic ointment to the site of venous catheterization—A controlled trial. *J Infect Dis* 120:611.

Page BH, Raine G, Jones PF. 1952. Thrombophelebitis following intravenous infusions. *Lancet* 2:778.

Performance of a New Softening Expanding Midline Catheter in Home Intravenous Therapy Patients. Journal of Intravenous Nursing, Vol. 14, No. 2 March/April '91. J.B. Lippincott Co.

Plumer A. 1982. *Principles and Practice of Intravenous Therapy,* 3ʳᵈ ed. Boston: Little, Brown.

Pollack M, Charache P, Nieman RE, et al. 1972. Factors influencing colonization and antibiotic-resistant patterns of gram-negative bacteria in hospital patients. *Lancet* 2:668.

Sager DP, Bomar SK. 1980. *Intravenous Medications: A Guide to Preparation, Administration, and Nursing Management.* Philadelphia: Lippincott.

Salzman TC, Clark JJ, Klemm L. 1967. Hand contamination of personnel as a mechanism of cross-infection in nosocomial infection with antibiotic-resistant Escherichia coil and Klebsiella aerobacter. *Antimicrob Agents Chemother* 97.

Sanderson I, Deitel M. 1973. Intravenous hyperalimentation without sepsis. *Surg Gynecol Obstet* 136:577.

Seiwin S, Ellis H. 1972. Skin bacteria and skin disinfection reconsidered. *Br Med J* 1:136.

Strumpher A. 1991. Lower Incidence of Peripheral Catheter Complications by Use of Elastomeric Hydrogel Catheters in Home Intravenous Therapy Patients. *J Intravenous Nursing* 14:4.

White JJ, Wallace CK, Burnett LS: Skin disinfection. *Johns Hopkins Med J* 126:169, 1970

Wilmore DW, Groff DB, Bishop HC, et al. 1969. Total parenteral nutrition in infants with catastrophic gastrointestinal anomalies. *J Pediatr Surg* 4:181.

Zinner SH, Denny-Brown BC, Braun P, et al. 1969. Risk of infection with intravenous indwelling catheters: Effective application of antibiotic ointment. *J Infect Dis* 120:616.

INDEX

sodium chloride (NaCl)   83, 147, 199-
     200 *see also* saline solution
solutes   141, 185
solution
     definition   185
     colored   148
     commonly used   199
     disposal   155
     quality   195
     tonicity   195
solvent   185
spiking   47-8, 130
spiking and priming, procedure   47, 49
splint   22-4
Sterile insertion tray   83, 89
sterile technique, using   85, 91, 95,
     97, 102, 104, 201
stimuli   21, 30
stopcock
     attachment   43, 112-13
     changing   153
     contamination source   43, 153-4,
          162, 218
stylet   63-7, 85, 137
Sublimation   275
superficial fascia   30
superior vena cava   87, 93-4, 96, 99,
     101, 103-4, 203
supplements *see* nutrition
support   279
swab, components   45
swabstick, use   84, 91, 95
Symbolization   275
synergistic effect   245, 250, 254
systemic circulation   18-19
SYSTEMIC PROBLEMS   165, 169-70

T

taping, methods   24, 72, 74-6
tapping   58
thrombitic occlusion, treatment   112
thrombophlebitis
     description   53, 163, 167
     intervention   164
     suppurative   164, 167

thrombosis   88, 95, 98, 102, 106, 204
thrombus, health hazard   20, 161
tissues
     damage   141, 155, 160
     elastic   21
     sclerosis of   102-3
titer   171, 224-5
TLC (triple lumen catheter)   99
tonicity   185, 195
total parenteral nutrition (TPN)
     administration   202
     complications   203
     definition   201
     duration   202
     indications   201
     therapy   203, 206-7
     using a filter   120
tourniquet   38, 55, 57-8, 64-5, 69, 76,
     78, 83-5, 88-9, 91-2, 95-6, 133,
     136, 158-9, 169
TPN *see* total parenteral nutrition
TPN pumps, programming   119
transfusion, monitoring   179
transparent semipermeable
          membrane (TSM)   73-6, 94, 96
tremors   188, 190
Trendelenburg position   33, 168
TSM *see* Transparent Semipermeable
          Membrane
tubing
     change   80, 152, 168, 205
     lipid   208
     piggyback   126
tunica intima   20
tunica media   20-1
Twin-Cath   40

U

U method, taping   75
Ultra Sound   85, 95

V

Valium   146, 148
valves   19-21, 49, 52

Lightning Source UK Ltd.
Milton Keynes UK
06 April 2011
170449UK00002B/15/P